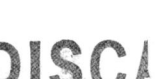

MW01603000

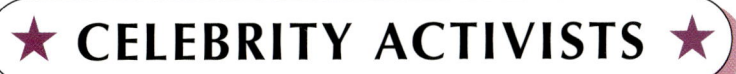

★ CELEBRITY ACTIVISTS ★

MEDICAL CAUSES

TANYA LEE STONE

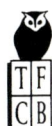

Twenty-First Century Books

A Division of Henry Holt and Company

New York

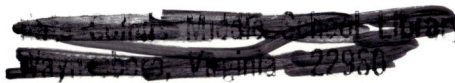

Twenty-First Century Books
A Division of Henry Holt and Company, Inc.
115 West 18th Street
New York, New York 10011

Henry Holt® and colophon are registered trademarks of Henry Holt and
Company, Inc.
Publishers since 1866

Published in Canada by Fitzhenry & Whiteside Ltd.
195 Allstate Parkway, Markham, Ontario L3R 4T8

Printed in the United States of America on acid free paper.∞

Created and produced in association with Blackbirch Graphics, Inc.

Library of Congress Cataloging-in-Publication Data

Stone, Tanya Lee
    Medical causes / Tanya Lee Stone.
        p.   cm. – (Celebrity activists)
    Includes bibliographical references and index.
    Summary: Features celebrities who have made major commitments
to helping others by contributing their time, money, and names for a
variety of medical causes.
    ISBN 0-8050-5233-X
    1. Medicine–Research–Endowments–Juvenile Literature. 2.
Celebrities–Charitable contributions. 3. Medical care–Endowments–
Juvenile literature. 4. Fund raisers (Persons)–Juvenile literature.
[1. Celebrities. 2. Fund raisers (Persons). 3. Medicine–Research.
4. Medical care.] I. Title.   II. Series.
R852.S76   1997
610'.7973–dc21   9725244
                                                                          CIP
                                                                           AC

CONTENTS

INTRODUCTION

One of our finest American traditions is philanthropy—giving of ourselves, by either donating time or money, to those who need us. Helping the less fortunate is part of our heritage and is a quality that we can be proud of.

For many people who are very well known to the public, this sense of responsibility toward others is especially strong. Successful athletes, actors, musicians, business leaders, and others often accept their positions in the spotlight as role models, and they look for opportunities to give something back to their communities. These celebrities play important roles in helping charitable groups educate the public and raise money for a variety of causes. When a favorite baseball player or movie star asks people for their help in benefiting a cause, chances are good that people are going to listen to the message and want to show their support.

There are thousands of nonprofit organizations in the United States that are working to improve our quality of life—whether it is by ending hunger and child abuse, protecting the environment, increasing literacy and educational opportunities, or helping to provide treatments and find cures for diseases.

In 1989, I established the Celebrity Outreach Foundation to help charitable groups enlist the help of celebrities who support their causes and are looking for opportunities to help. It was the first organization of its kind in the country. To date, we have matched more than 600 celebrities with 350 nonprofit organizations.

Before we could help anyone, however, we had to establish our own credibility as a new foundation. Gregory Peck, Whoopi Goldberg, Dan Aykroyd, Eddie Murphy, Alec Baldwin, Tony Danza, and others stepped forward to support our efforts. A Celebrity Advisory Committee was formed. The names of all the committee members are featured in our promotion materials. Without the committee's support, it would have been much more difficult to establish our identity.

The celebrities featured in this book have all made major commitments by contributing their time, money, and names to help a variety of causes. (There are many others, but unfortunately we do not have the space to include every philanthropic celebrity.) Their efforts have made a significant difference in the lives of many people.

Bob Oettinger
Celebrity Outreach Foundation

DISEASES THAT AFFECT CHILDREN

Pediatrics is the name of the branch of medicine that focuses on babies and children. That is why a doctor for children is called a pediatrician. There are many diseases that affect both children and adults. Since children may experience the same disease differently than grownups do, they are often treated separately. For example, diabetes can begin in childhood (Type I diabetes) or in adulthood (Type II diabetes). When a child has diabetes, it is often referred to as "juvenile diabetes." Other diseases, such as muscular dystrophy, afflict mainly children.

Some people who become involved with medical causes focus their efforts specifically on helping children and their families. That is what all the stories in this chapter share in common. Organizations such as the Juvenile Diabetes Foundation, the Starlight Children's Foundation, and the Muscular Dystrophy Association dedicate themselves to improving patient care and funding important research for childhood diseases. In this way, they make a dramatic impact on the lives of children around the world.

★ Paul Newman ★

Throughout his career, Paul Newman has starred in dozens of movies. In 1986, he won an Academy Award for *The Color of Money*. In addition to being known as a great movie star, Newman is recognized as a first-class philanthropist.

In 1982, Newman and a friend of his, A.E. Hotchner, founded Newman's Own, Inc. Their intention was to sell salad dressing made from the actor's own recipe and distribute the profits to charity. The salad dressing sold so well that the company soon offered popcorn, lemonade, and spaghetti sauce. Today, the company is thriving. At the end of each year, Newman reviews funding applications from a variety of organizations that are looking for contributions. Newman gives away every penny of the company's after-tax profits—now about $10 million a year.

In the early years of Newman's Own, among the requests for help that the company received were dozens of letters from parents of children who had cancer. Newman's heart went out to these children and their families. In 1986, he came up with an idea that would make a huge difference in their lives. His dream took shape in the form of The Hole in the Wall Gang Camp, named after the Hole in the Wall Gang in his movie *Butch Cassidy and the Sundance Kid*.

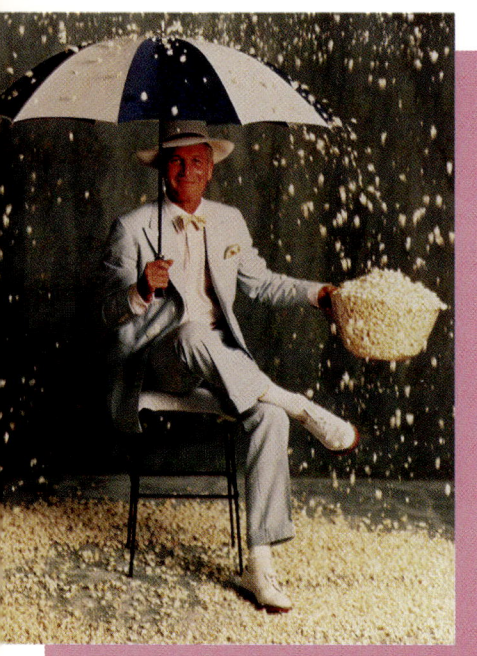

Paul Newman donates all of the after-tax profits from Newman's Own, Inc. to charity.

This nonprofit summer camp is for children with cancer and life-threatening blood diseases. Each year, free of charge, 900 children between the ages of 7 and 15 live at the camp. They fish, hike, swim, ride horses, and play tennis, softball, or basketball. This camp does wonders for kids who are usually confined to a life of hospital stays and doctor's visits. Their experiences at the camp help them to stay joyous and hopeful in the face of life-threatening illnesses.

Everything about The Hole in the Wall Gang Camp is extraordinary. Even though it is equipped with all the necessary medical equipment and round-the-clock personnel needed, it is all disguised. Campers are barely aware that they are staying at a top-notch medical facility. When the kids first arrive, they see a camp in the middle of 300 acres of forest. It looks like a frontier town, with some important, though scarcely noticeable, differences. Walkways end in access ramps. Forest trails are smooth and wide enough for wheelchairs. The log cabins that house campers are arranged in a circle with a center that is large enough for helicopter transport to land in an emergency. The infirmary sign reads "The O.K. Corrall"—named by a camper "because it's okay to go there."

Dr. Howard Pearson, professor of pediatrics at Yale University and former president of the American Academy of Pediatrics, has been the medical director of the camp from the start. Pearson lives at the camp in the summer. He also serves on the camp's

Medical Advisory Board of physicians. One of the most important jobs of the board is to decide how to best care for the medical needs of campers.

It cost $17 million to build this Connecticut camp, which opened in 1988. Newman donated over $8 million from Newman's Own profits to start the camp. Both large and small volunteer groups raised the rest of the money. Volunteers from the U.S. Navy built a footbridge, floating dock, and trails. School groups held car washes, and construction services were donated by a local developer named Simon Konover. These were only a few of the early participants. The $2 million per year it takes to run this camp is successfully raised by generous group and individual contributors across the country. Newman continues to be an active force in The Hole in the Wall Gang Camp. He is president of the organization, and is always around for a day or two during each camp session, interacting with the kids.

In addition to the work he accomplishes through Newman's Own and The Hole in the Wall Gang Camp, Paul Newman works for other causes. He and his wife Joanne Woodward established the Scott Newman Foundation in memory of their son, who died in 1978. The foundation, centered in Los Angeles, provides drug education and runs an addiction recovery program. Newman is also a major contributor to the Big Apple Circus Clown Care Unit. This is a group of specially trained clowns dedicated to spreading joy among sick children. In fact, the clowns comfort and entertain Hole in the Wall Gang campers when needed. They even provide the camp with a resident clown. Through the generosity and spirit of Paul Newman, thousands of kids are helped and hundreds of volunteers have an incredible opportunity to make a difference.

★ *Jerry Lewis* ★

Jerry Lewis is one of the most famous comedians in the world. He is also one of the best-known philanthropists. In 1950, Lewis started raising funds for the newly formed Muscular Dystrophy Association (MDA). The MDA was founded to help children who suffered from neuromuscular diseases—diseases that affect the muscles and nerves. Many people think that muscular dystrophy is one disease, but there are actually nine different kinds. There are also 31 other diseases that affect the muscles and nerves. The MDA focuses on all 40 of these illnesses. As time went on, Lewis's personal commitment to the Muscular Dystrophy Association grew.

In 1966, Lewis began the annual Jerry Lewis "Stars Across America!" Labor Day Telethon—a marathon fund-raising event in which people call in to pledge money for the MDA. The first year, only one station aired the telethon, but the event made history. It was the first televised fund-raiser to raise over $1 million. Over the years, the telethon grew. By 1970, it was carried by 65 stations. Today, 200 stations across the country broadcast the telethon, which has raised over $800 million for the MDA. The money supports research and helps provide medical and other services for patients and families. Some of the telethon money also goes toward educational efforts, so that patients, families, and the general public can be better informed about neuromuscular diseases. Throughout the year, Lewis fulfills his duties as the MDA national chairman. He visits with children who suffer from neuromuscular diseases, appeals to corporations for donations, and attends meetings with scientists who are looking for treatments and cures.

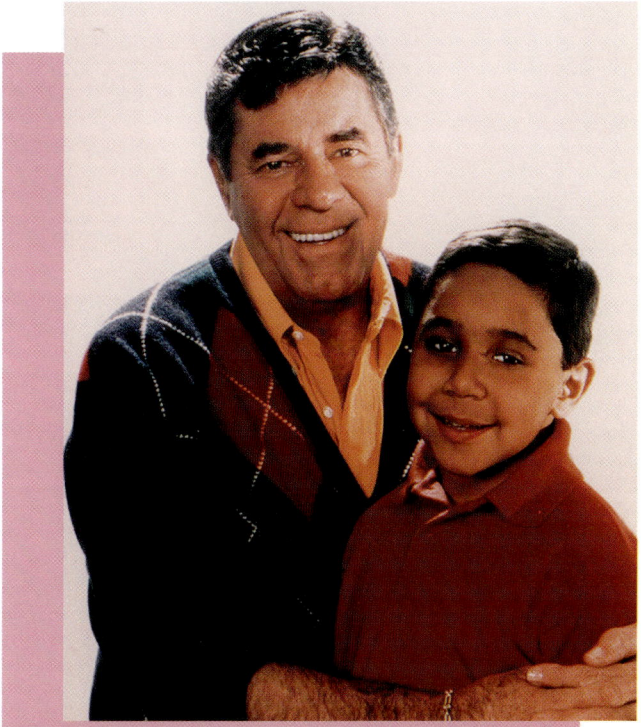

Since 1950, Lewis (shown here with National Goodwill Ambassador Benjamin Cumbo) has been dedicated to the MDA.

In addition to Jerry Lewis, many other celebrities hold important volunteer positions at the MDA, including Ed McMahon, Ann-Margret, Maureen McGovern, Magic Johnson, Wynton Marsalis, and Casey Kasem. McMahon, who has anchored the telethon for more than 20 years, said of Lewis, "Through TV, [Lewis] was able to . . . communicate the urgency and hope offered by research, to show his endless love for 'his kids,' and to introduce millions of viewers to people with disabilities with an emphasis on their abilities, their strengths, and their humanity. . . . No single performer is so closely associated with a particular humanitarian cause as is Jerry Lewis."

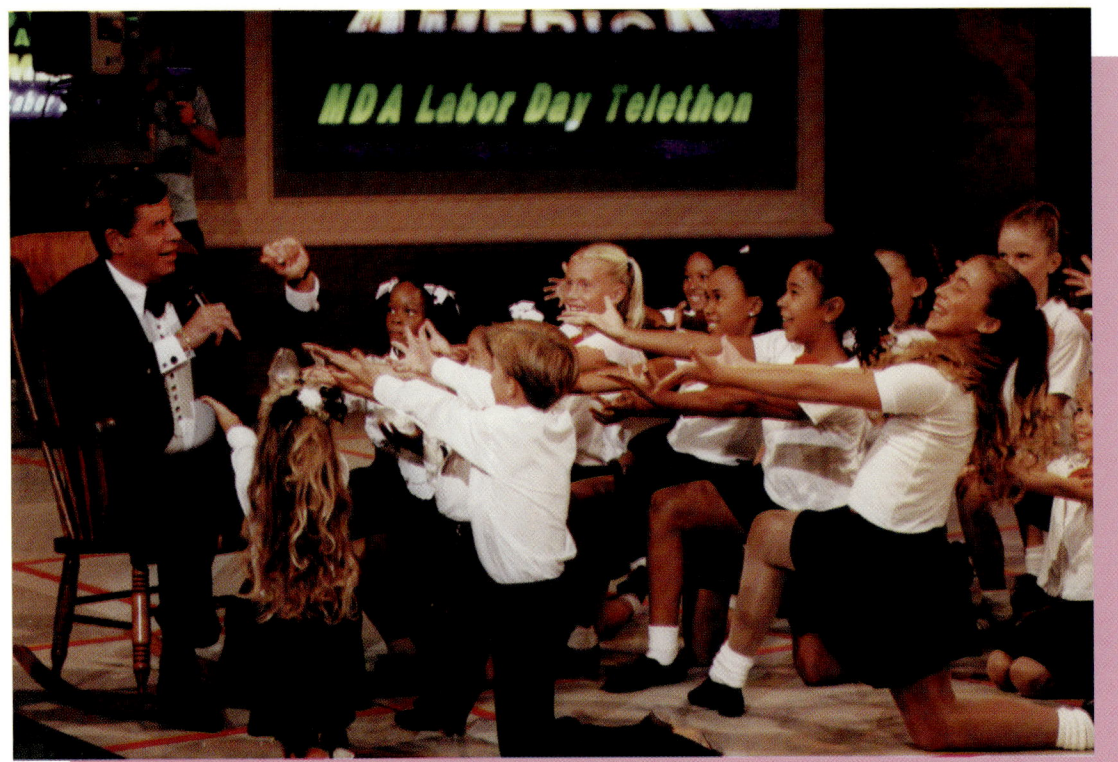

Jerry Lewis performs with the Anita Mann Dancers during the 1996 telethon.

Lewis has been honored many times for his work with the MDA. In 1977, he was nominated for a Nobel Peace Prize, which was the only time an entertainer has ever been nominated. In 1984, he was admitted into the French Legion of Honor and made a Commander in the Order of Arts and Letters. The French Minister of Culture, Jack Lang, told Lewis, "You are a child's friend, and a model for adults." In 1985, the U.S. Defense Department gave Lewis its highest civilian award—the Medal for Distinguished Public Service.

Lewis's feelings toward his philanthropic work are reflected by this quotation, which is close to his heart: "I shall pass through this world but once. Any good, therefore, that I can do or any kindness that I can show to any human being, let me do it now. Let me not defer nor neglect, for I shall not pass this way again."

The Starlight Children's Foundation

The Starlight Children's Foundation was established in 1983 by actress Emma Samms and film executive Peter Samuelson. The foundation began when these two cousins were lucky enough to meet a boy named Sean, who changed their lives. Sean was very ill, and he had always wanted to go to Disney World. Emma and Peter decided to grant his wish and pay for Sean's trip. They were overwhelmed by how it made them feel to be able to bring him some joy.

Starlight's mission is to brighten the lives of seriously ill children. The way they do this is through activities for both children who are in the hospital and those who are able to stay at home but are also very sick. Starlight is an international, nonprofit organization that helps as many as 43,000 children each month! Starlight reaches these kids through three main programs—Fun Centers, Wish-Granting, and Starlight Rooms.

Starlight's Fun Centers are mobile entertainment units that are wheeled into the rooms of hospitalized children. The units fit right over their beds. Each Fun Center has a VCR, television monitor, Nintendo Game system, and game cartridges. There are over 12,000 Fun

Centers in 540 hospitals worldwide. They are paid for with the help of Nintendo of America and other corporate sponsors.

Some hospitals also have Starlight Rooms, where state-of-the-art media facilities are provided for both children who stay at the hospital and children who have to go there often for special care. This unique environment encourages kids to be creative and gives them a break from thinking about their illnesses. These rooms let them have fun right in the hospital!

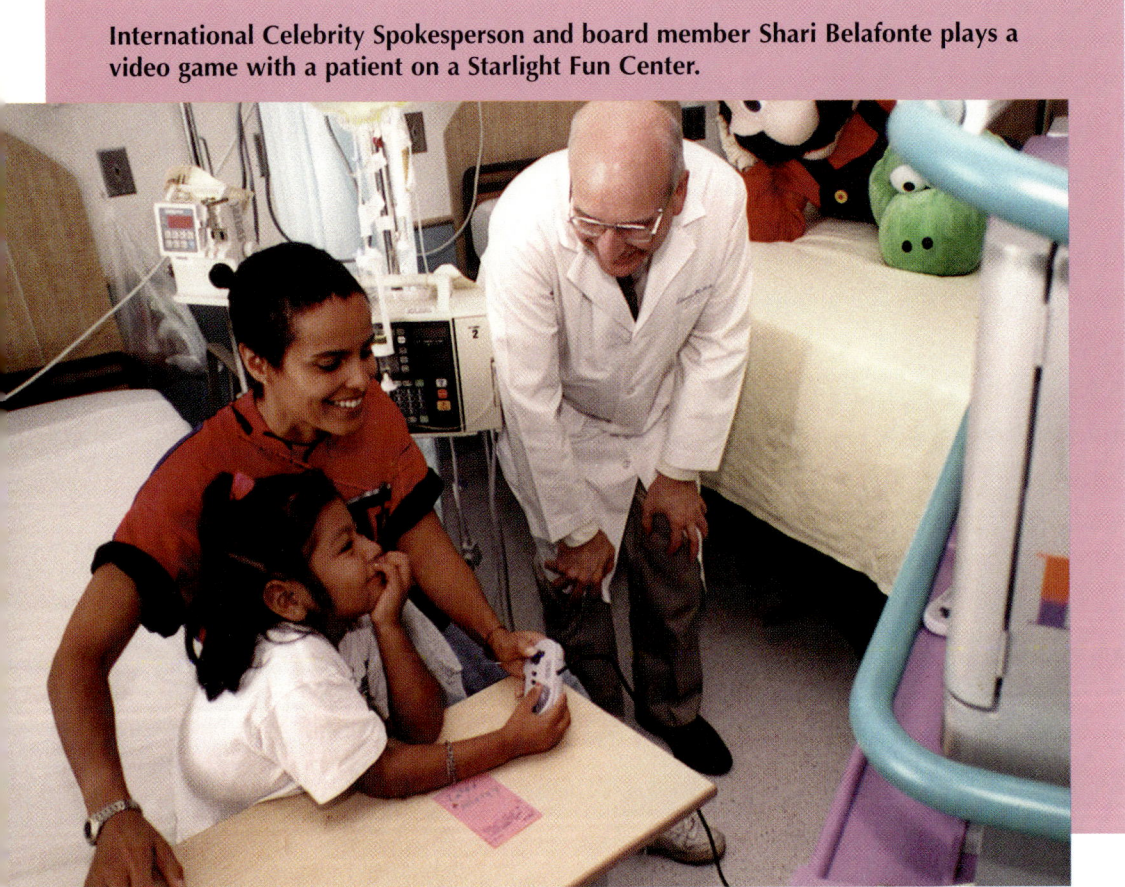

International Celebrity Spokesperson and board member Shari Belafonte plays a video game with a patient on a Starlight Fun Center.

In 1995, Starlight reached a landmark after granting the 14,000th wish through their Wish-Granting program. Starlight works tirelessly to make the dreams of these very special children come true. For example, a 12-year-old girl got to meet Michael Jordan, and a 15-year-old boy was sent to the 1996 Summer Olympics. Starlight's special children are most commonly afflicted with one of the following diseases: leukemia, kidney disease, cystic fibrosis, muscular dystrophy, spina bifida, cerebral palsy, and pediatric AIDS.

As Starlight has grown, many corporate sponsors, or business donors, have generously contributed services, products, and money to help fund the organization. These include American Airlines, Nintendo of America, Toys "R" Us, Wal-Mart, and Colgate-Palmolive. Many celebrities support Starlight in a variety of ways, such as attending events, granting wishes, or donating autographed items. Sail With The Stars®—an annual cruise during which families interact with teen celebrities—donates its on-board profits to Starlight. Each year at the Annual Daytime Stars for Starlight event, many soap opera stars donate their time and help to grant Starlight wishes. And the fX network held a Personal fX Science Fiction Auction and donated all of the proceeds to Starlight. Gabrielle Carteris, of "Beverly Hills 90210," is featured in a public service announcement for Starlight on CBS. Starlight's current celebrity spokespeople are Shari Belafonte, Tori Spelling, Cheryl Ladd, and Shirley Jones.

Danny Thomas

The St. Jude Children's Research Hospital, founded by Danny Thomas, specializes in helping children who are very ill.

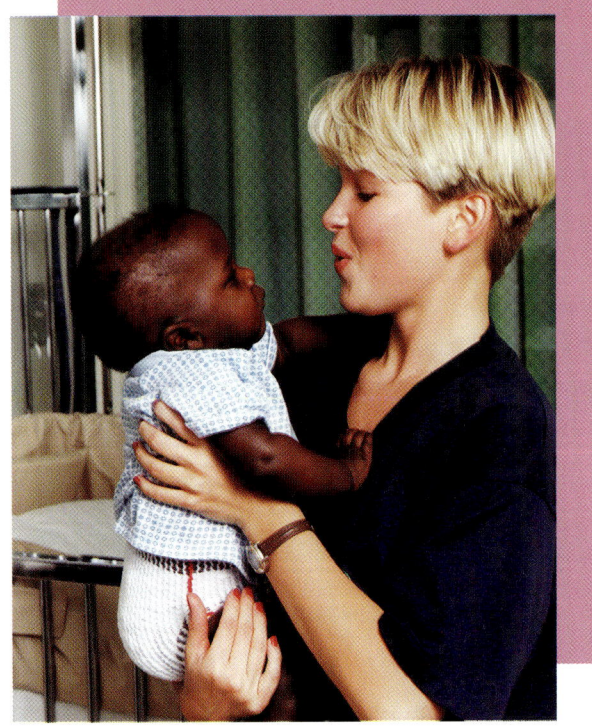

When Danny Thomas was a struggling comedian, he prayed to St. Jude, the patron saint of impossible, hopeless, and difficult causes. In his prayers, he said to St. Jude "[if you will help me] find my place in life, I will build you a shrine where the poor, helpless, and hopeless may come for comfort and aid." He fulfilled that promise when he founded the St. Jude Children's Research Hospital in Memphis, Tennessee. Opened in 1962, it is now the largest childhood cancer research center in America.

The children who are helped at St. Jude Hospital are victims

of some of the most debili-
tating childhood diseases—
Hodgkin disease, leukemia,
and other cancers, as well as
sickle-cell disease. Patients
are admitted to St. Jude Hospital because they suffer
from diseases that are being
studied at this research center. It is the first center that
was created strictly for the
purpose of researching cata-
strophic childhood diseases,
and it is staffed by some of
the finest doctors in the
world. One of them,
Dr. Peter Doherty, even

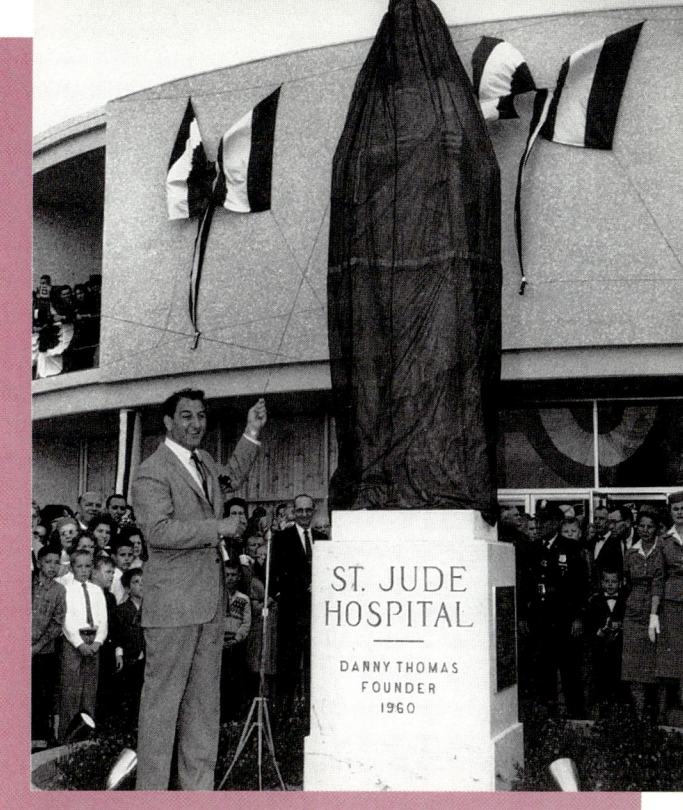

**Danny Thomas prepares to unveil a statue of St.
Jude at the 1962 opening of the hospital.**

received a Nobel Prize for his work on the immune system.

Thomas, who died in 1992, dedicated his life to raising the
money needed to operate the hospital's research and treatment
programs. He established a national fund-raising organization
called the American Lebanese Syrian Associated Charities (ALSAC).
St. Jude Hospital receives most of its financial support from contributions raised by ALSAC. The research hospital is also funded
by grants from the National Institutes of Health (NIH) and the
National Cancer Institute.

One special feature of St. Jude Hospital is that no patient is
ever asked to pay. Any costs not covered by insurance are paid by
St. Jude Hospital and ALSAC—they even pay the lodging and
travel expenses for the patient and one parent.

★ *Mary Tyler Moore* ★

The actress Mary Tyler Moore found her way into America's heart first as Laura Petrie on "The Dick Van Dyke Show," and then as Mary Richards on "The Mary Tyler Moore Show." With her former husband, Grant Tinker, Moore formed a successful production company called M.T.M. She has since gone on to star in movies and on Broadway.

Moore has lived with juvenile diabetes for much of her life. Diabetes is a defect in insulin metabolism. Insulin is what allows sugars to be broken down so that the body's cells can make energy. In juvenile diabetes, there is a lack of insulin because the cells that normally produce it are defective. (In people who develop diabetes as adults, there is a decrease in the amount of insulin produced.) Diabetes affects up to 120 million people worldwide and about 16 million Americans. Complications from this disease include kidney failure, heart disease, stroke, blindness, and loss of nerve function.

For the past 12 years, Moore has been the International Chairman of the Juvenile Diabetes Foundation (JDF) International. This organization was founded in 1970. Its primary goal is to fund diabetes research. Through research, doctors and scientists find cures for diseases. In Moore's view, "Whether you're looking for a way to turn electricity into light, or to find a cure for diabetes, there's no way of knowing what will and won't work without research....And research will find a cure for diabetes—if we have the will and determination to sustain that research with adequate financial support."

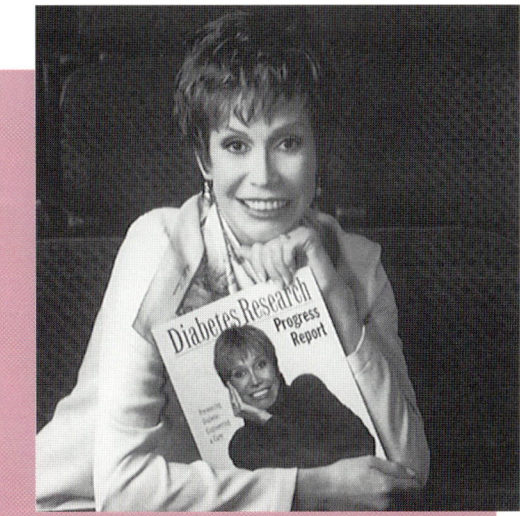

Mary Tyler Moore has been the International Chairman of the JDF for 12 years.

Since 1970, JDF has raised more than $200 million to benefit diabetes research. This research has not always been given the financial attention it needs. Some people mistakenly think the treatment for diabetes—insulin injections—is a cure. But insulin is just a treatment.

Moore is always at the disposal of JDF to give whatever help it needs. She has testified before Congressional committees on behalf of the organization. She has appeared in numerous public service announcements, television programs, and fund-raising events. She serves as the co-chairman of JDF's The Only Remedy Is a Cure fund-raising campaign. Moore also donates a large amount of the profits from her exercise video to JDF.

Money that is raised for JDF is awarded to doctors and scientists who apply for grants to fund their research. JDF donates more money directly to diabetes research than any other private health agency in the world. Individual chapters of JDF also offer support groups for families with children who are affected by juvenile diabetes. Moore's commitment to JDF has helped to raise public awareness of this disease.

THE BATTLE AGAINST AIDS

AIDS stands for acquired immune deficiency syndrome. The virus that causes this disease is called HIV—the human immunodeficiency virus. HIV is spread in a number of ways, including through sexual activity between an infected person and someone who is healthy. People also acquire AIDS by sharing needles and syringes. Most people who get AIDS this way are drug users, but there have been a few cases of health-care workers who have accidentally nicked themselves and become ill. Someone can also get AIDS through blood transfusions or organ transplants. The risk of this happening today is very low because blood is now screened for the virus. A pregnant woman infected with HIV can transmit the disease to her baby. It is not possible, however, to transmit this virus via drinking glasses, kissing, coughing, sneezing, touching, by using a toilet seat, or swimming in a pool.

AIDS affects millions of people around the world—both adults and children. Money for adequate patient care is needed, as is funding for continued research that will hopefully bring us closer to a cure. All of the people in this chapter are dedicated to improving patient care and furthering research efforts.

Elizabeth Taylor

In 1992, Elizabeth Taylor, one of the most famous movie stars in the world, established the Elizabeth Taylor AIDS Foundation (ETAF). She created this foundation to fund AIDS organizations around the world that provide patient care, support services, and prevention education programs. In doing so, Taylor became the first celebrity crusader for AIDS. Hers is one of the biggest AIDS organizations in the world. ETAF distributed almost $4.5 million in its first four years.

One of the unique things about this foundation is that Taylor personally pays for all of

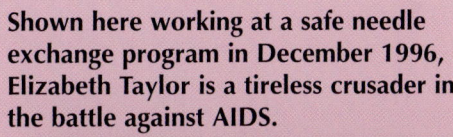

Shown here working at a safe needle exchange program in December 1996, Elizabeth Taylor is a tireless crusader in the battle against AIDS.

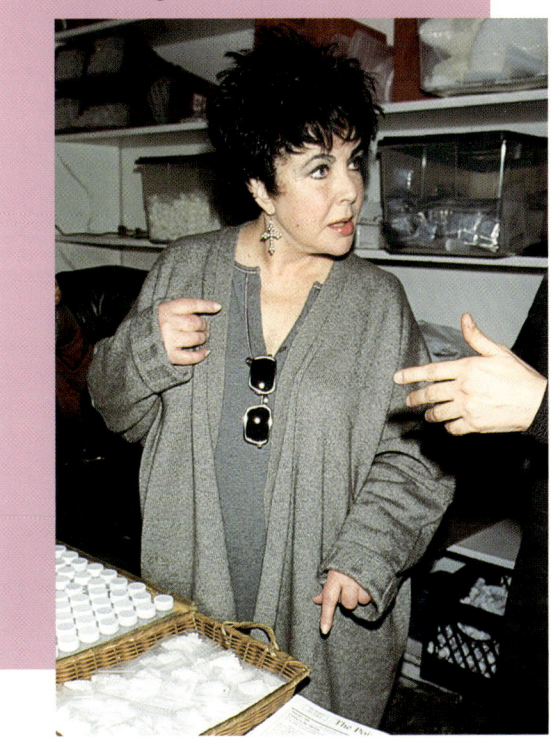

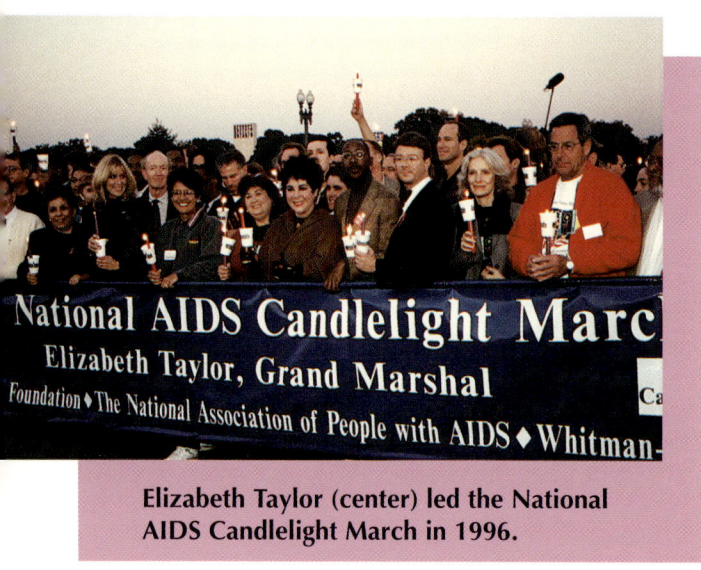

Elizabeth Taylor (center) led the National AIDS Candlelight March in 1996.

the costs associated with running it. These costs include paying staff, putting on benefit events, and printing promotional materials. This means that every cent that is donated to the Elizabeth Taylor AIDS Foundation is put directly toward helping people with HIV and AIDS live as comfortably as possible.

ETAF has awarded grants to many AIDS service organizations, including AIDS Project Los Angeles, the American Foundation for AIDS Research (AmFAR), New Mexico AIDS Services, Rhode Island AIDS Project, Utah AIDS Foundation, People of Color Against AIDS Network, Minority AIDS Project, and Caring for Babies with AIDS.

Taylor is constantly toiling in the fight against AIDS. In October 1996, she led the National AIDS Candlelight March. In December 1996, she volunteered her time to work with patients in a needle exchange program in New York City. She also speaks out in favor of safe sex and teen abstinence. She gave a speech on these subjects at the National Press Club in Washington, D.C., in July 1996. In February 1997, a celebration of Taylor's 65th birthday was the focus of a major fund-raiser to benefit the Elizabeth Taylor AIDS Foundation. The star-studded event was held at the Pantages Theatre in Hollywood and raised more than $1 million for the organization. At the benefit, Madonna spoke about Taylor's work for AIDS saying, "Elizabeth Taylor has stopped making films, but her life continues to shine in a much more wondrous passion."

Elton John

Although you may have never heard of Reginald Kenneth Dwight, the singer who became known as Elton John is famous throughout the world. By the mid-1970s, John played concerts that sold out to crowds of over 100,000, was on the cover of *Time* magazine, had a hit record with the late Beatles singer John Lennon, and had his own star on the Hollywood Walk of Fame. In the 1980s, he and his music partner, Bernie Taupin, had a string of hits. From the beginning, he was flamboyant on stage. John dyed his hair countless times and dressed in the most outrageous costumes imaginable.

In the late 1980s, Elton John had an experience that changed his life forever. He became friends with Ryan White, a high school student who was barred from his Indiana school because he had contracted AIDS from a blood transfusion. White went to court to be allowed to return to school, and won his case in 1990. Soon after, White died in the hospital, and Elton John was at his side. Two years later, John decided to donate all of his profits from his hit singles to AIDS. He founded the Elton John AIDS Foundation, which is now one of the world's largest AIDS organizations. John serves as its chairman.

The mission of the Elton John AIDS Foundation is to fund patient care and HIV/AIDS prevention and education. The non-profit international organization does not fund research, but it has made a huge impact on the quality of education and services available for the millions of people afflicted with HIV and AIDS. To date, the Elton John AIDS Foundation has raised more than $7.5 million. The money that is distributed each year supports services such as food banks, meal delivery programs, counseling, support groups, legal assistance, at-home care, education programs, and pediatric treatment centers.

Each year, the foundation organizes a variety of successful fund-raising events, often with the help of other celebrities. In 1993, Billie Jean King (who, along with Whoopi Goldberg, serves on the advisory board of the foundation) and John presented the first annual World TEAMTENNIS All Star Smash Hits® in Los Angeles. They raised $500,000. This event has been a success every year. Martina Navratilova, John McEnroe, Andre Agassi, Monica Seles, and Pete Sampras have each joined in the fun. Another annual event sponsored by Elton John that raises hundreds of thousands of dollars for the foundation is the annual Academy Awards Viewing Party, which also began in 1993. Stars such as Sylvester Stallone, Bruce Springsteen, Steven Spielberg, Tom Hanks, Sharon Stone, Robin Williams, Michael Douglas, and many others support this event each year.

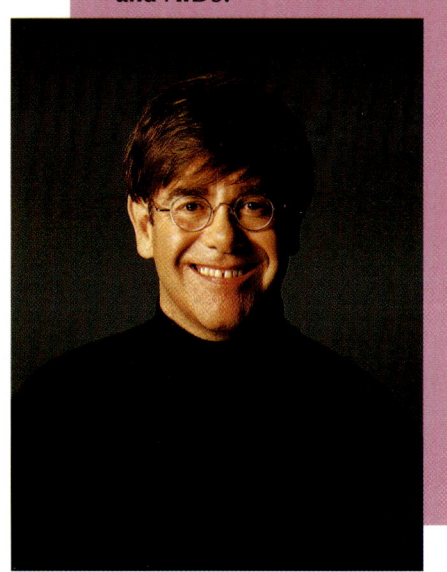

Through his foundation, Elton John has helped educate people about HIV and AIDS.

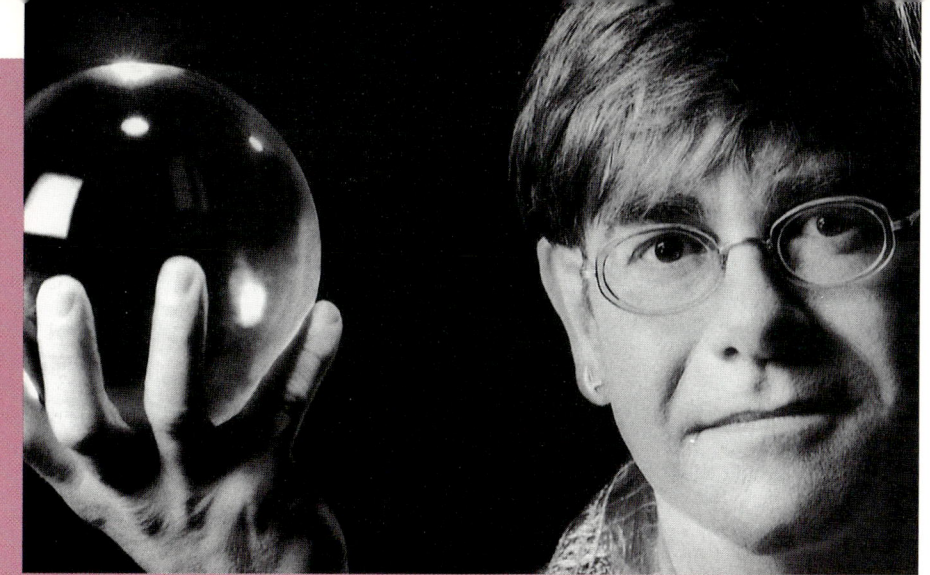

In a promotion piece for the foundation, Elton John asks us to "share our vision for a better future."

The number of events that Elton John hosts throughout each year is staggering. In 1995 and 1996, John literally cleaned out his closets and donated hundreds of his own outfits to a benefit called Elton's Closet. All of the sale money went to the foundation. John says of the event, "Most people know by now that I love clothes, and I certainly have enough closets to part with some of my favorite things and still have enough to wear!" Other inspired fund-raisers include the 1993 and 1995 sale of signature series Hard Rock Cafe T-shirts. In 1995, the T-shirt design was a self-portrait by the musician Sting. The donations for the foundation from those two events totaled more than $1.2 million.

John says of the foundation, "I have spoken publicly about my personal fight against the addictions that almost cost me my life. I have spoken of my gratitude at being given a second chance and my wish to give something back to society. I have lost many friends to AIDS, and I know so many more who are living with HIV and AIDS....It continues to be a ...battle....There is room on the battlefield for all of us and each and every one of you is needed....I invite you to join me in the fight."

Paul Michael and Elizabeth Glaser

Paul Michael Glaser is probably best known as an actor for his role as Starsky on the detective show "Starsky and Hutch." He is now a successful director and an AIDS crusader. In 1981, when his wife Elizabeth was delivering their first child, she needed a blood transfusion. This was at a time when AIDS was still considered rare in the United States. Doctors did not realize that many of the nation's blood supplies might be contaminated with the virus. Four years later, however, the Glasers' young daughter Ariel became very sick. Eventually, the whole family was tested for HIV. Paul tested negative, but Elizabeth tested positive. She had contracted HIV through the blood transfusions she had received, and she had passed the virus on to Ariel. At the time the Glasers received this information, Elizabeth was pregnant with their second child, Jake. The virus had, unfortunately, also been passed on to him.

When Ariel was just seven years old, she died of AIDS. This tragedy affected the Glasers deeply. They wanted to try and make sure that no other parents would experience this pain. In 1988, Elizabeth made a plea to Congress to increase funding for AIDS research. She also met with former president Ronald Reagan and his wife, Nancy. Partly as a

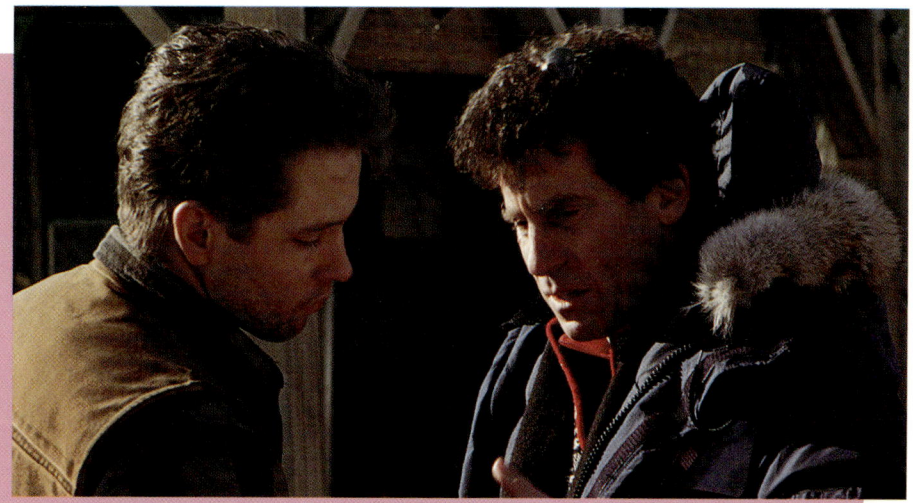

Director Paul Michael Glaser (right) continues to play an active role in the Pediatric AIDS Foundation.

result of her efforts, the federal budget for AIDS was raised from $3.3 to $8.8 million.

Elizabeth founded the Pediatric AIDS Foundation in 1988 with two friends, Susan DeLaurentis and Susie Zeegen. Together, they created the only organization dedicated exclusively to funding research for children with AIDS. In the first eight months, the foundation raised $2.2 million and funded 40 research grants.

In July 1992, Elizabeth gave a speech at the Democratic National Convention. In it, she urged the government to step up its efforts toward caring for people with AIDS. She spoke of the prejudice that surrounds people who suffer from this disease, and she noted the need for a national leader committed to educating people. She said, "We need a visionary to guide us—to say it *wasn't* all right for Ryan White to be banned from school because he had HIV....Do you know how much my AIDS care

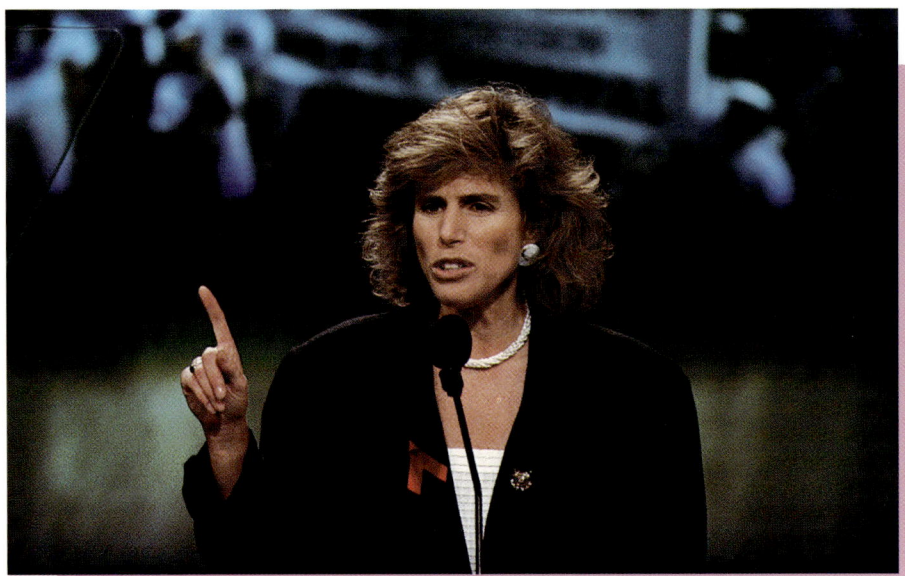

Elizabeth Glaser addresses delegates at the 1992 Democratic Convention.

costs? More than $40,000 a year. Someone without insurance can't afford this.... This is not the America I was raised to be proud of—where the rich people get care and drugs that poor people can't. We need health care for all. We need a leader to say this, and do something about it."

Elizabeth Glaser died in December 1994. Her son Jake, although infected by HIV, has not shown any signs of developing AIDS. Paul Michael Glaser has been on the board of directors for the Pediatric AIDS Foundation for the last few years. He now works diligently for the same cause that his wife dedicated herself to. The foundation established the Elizabeth Glaser Scientist Award in her memory. Each year, it funds the research of up to five scientists who are committed to learning more about pediatric AIDS.

★ *Sharon Stone* ★

Sharon Stone is one of Hollywood's most popular actresses. She has also become one of the most visible activists of the entertainment industry. In December 1995, she was chosen as the chairman for the new fund-raising campaign created by the American Foundation for AIDS Research (AmFAR). She made a three-year commitment to the organization, vowing to help them reach their goal of raising $76 million for AIDS research.

AmFAR is America's leading nonprofit organization for AIDS research, education, and public policy. Research grants that have been funded by AmFAR have resulted in better diagnosis, prevention, and treatment of AIDS. The organization's education efforts ensure that patients and health-care professionals alike receive the latest information about the disease. AmFAR's public policy efforts strive to protect the rights of people with HIV/AIDS.

Stone's primary responsibility as chairman of AmFAR is to raise public awareness of the need for research on controlling the spread of HIV worldwide. While accepting this position at a World AIDS Day lunch she said, "[I am] honored to stand on the front lines beside compassionate and effective leaders in the fight against AIDS....I accepted to lead the campaign for AIDS research because I know that only research can justify and sustain the hope that we will vanquish AIDS." Stone has spoken at the United Nations and before Congress. She has also appeared at numerous AmFAR events since she became its chairman.

Sharon Stone meets with Samuel Kayman of the Public Health Research Institute of New York, whose research on an AIDS vaccine has been funded by AmFAR since 1993.

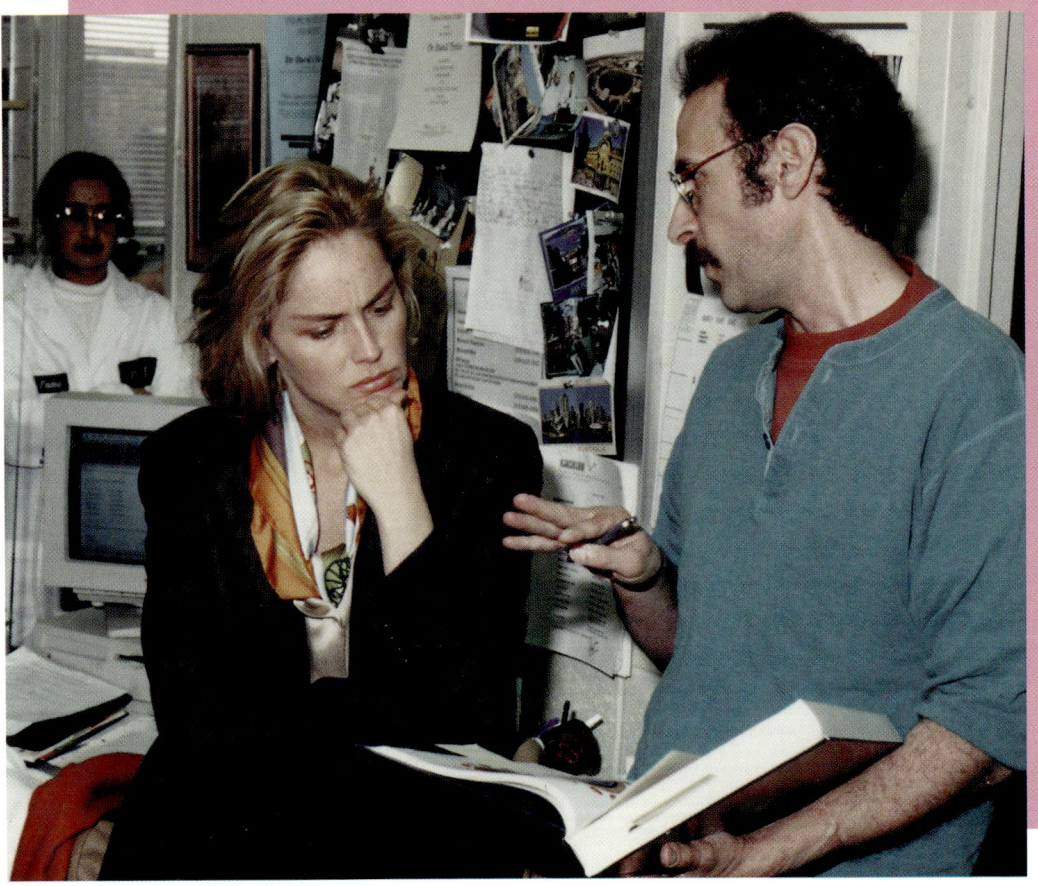

AmFAR
AIDS RESEARCH

AmFAR funds grants related to AIDS research and education.

In an interview on "Movieline" in September 1996, Stone was asked to describe her biggest accomplishment for AmFAR to date. She replied, "I think I've helped wake people up again. I've reminded them that they have a commitment to ending this disease, and that it is possible." Stone's attitude about fund-raising reflects her belief that people are often more generous than they think they are. She encourages everyone to get involved, not just those who can afford to make hefty contributions. In the "Movieline" interview she was asked what fans and supporters could do who are not rich. She responded, "Give me one dollar." And she has set up a mailing address through AmFAR for just that purpose. Stone's philosophy is one that many of the philanthropic celebrities in this book share. The overall message for people to understand is that by working together, no matter in what capacity, human beings can make an impact.

AmFAR is not the only organization to benefit from Stone's involvement. In 1991, Stone and her sister Kelly founded Planet Hope, an organization that helps provide job placement to homeless individuals and support to their families.

AIDS Project Los Angeles

AIDS Project Los Angeles (APLA) is a nonprofit group dedicated to improving the quality of life for Los Angeles County residents affected by HIV. APLA also provides education for people who are at-risk of contracting this virus. In order to reduce the incidence of people with HIV/AIDS, APLA fights for fair legislation on the local, state, and federal levels on behalf of people with AIDS. Founded in 1982, the group established the nation's first HIV/AIDS hotline—a telephone line staffed by volunteers who provide callers with information about AIDS. APLA has had significant celebrity support from the beginning.

Elizabeth Taylor gives her time by serving on the board of governors. She also worked for the annual fund-raiser called Commitment To Life (CTL). This event features a celebrity variety show and awards ceremony. The first benefit raised $1.3 million for the organization. Elton John has donated his talents to several past Commitment To Life events and was given a CTL award for his work in the battle against AIDS.

David Geffen, a major music producer, has been a generous donor since the group began. He contributed $1 million toward the purchase of APLA's headquarters and continues this support with an annual

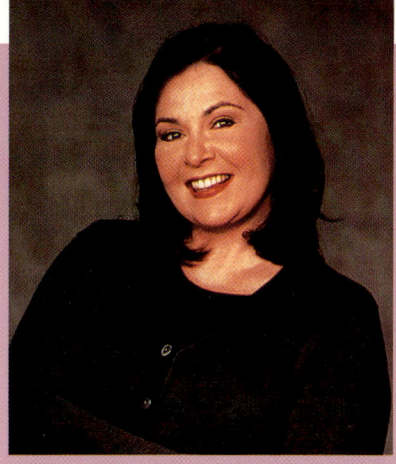
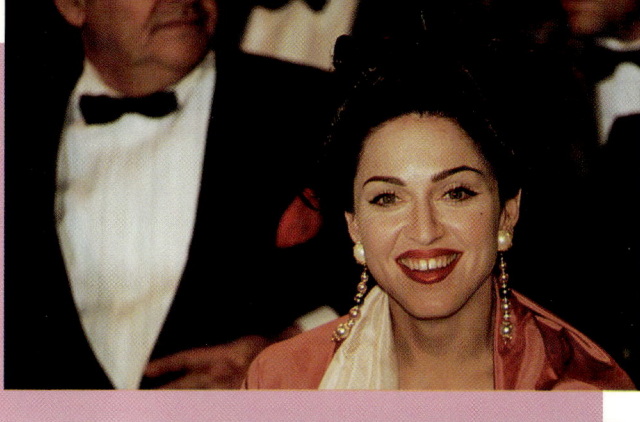
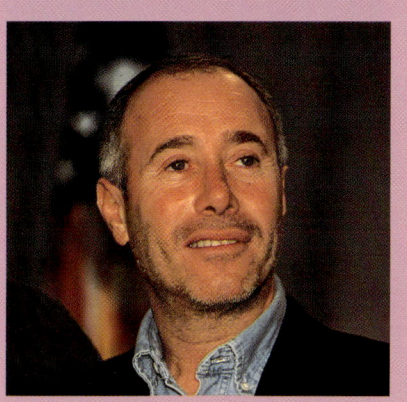
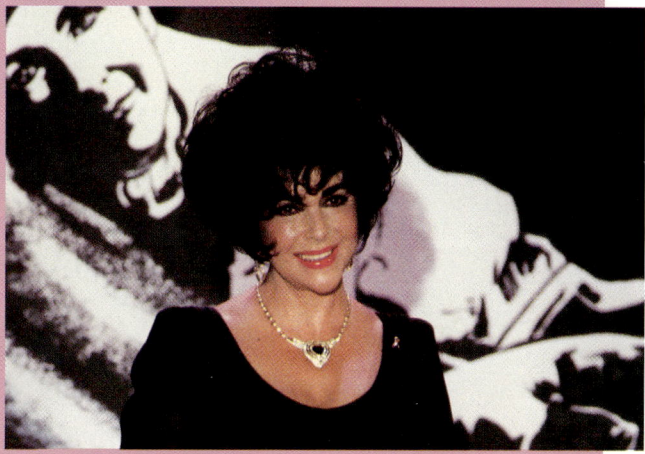

(Clockwise from upper left) Roseanne, Madonna, Elizabeth Taylor, and David Geffen are just a few of the stars who support AIDS Project Los Angeles.

donation of $250,000 toward the mortgage payment. APLA honored him for his contributions by naming the building The Geffen Center. Geffen has committed a significant amount of his time to the organization. He has served as a former board chair of APLA and continues to be a member of the board of governors. In addition, Geffen works as a committee co-chair for many of the Commitment To Life galas.

The actress Roseanne has also dedicated herself to APLA. She has helped on many occasions, hosting a benefit art show at The Geffen Center, participating in a 1995 tribute to Frank Sinatra for APLA, and appearing in the 1996 CTL. Madonna has also frequently made herself available to APLA. She has appeared in many of their events, including an AIDS Dance-A-Thon and several CTL evenings. The Dance-A-Thon is an annual event and some of the proceeds also benefit other Los Angeles AIDS organizations. The group Salt-N-Pepa has also donated their time by appearing in numerous APLA events.

The monies raised through all of the different APLA benefits fund about 20 different programs. These include: the Necessities of Life Food Pantry, providing $2 million of groceries for more than 1,600 people a year; the Buddy Program, offering emotional support and social interaction through telephone calls and home and hospital visits; the Southern California HIV/AIDS Hotline; Skills for Teen AIDS Risk Reduction, a program that educates thousands of high school students each year; and HIV Health Education Forums.

The number of celebrities that support APLA are too numerous to mention. It is clear that the entertainment industry believes wholeheartedly in fighting the battle against AIDS. Through the hard work and dedication of countless people, necessary funding for patient services and crucial research is raised each year.

People suffer from many different kinds of cancer. The most common forms you are likely to have heard about are breast, ovarian, lung, and skin cancer. But there are many others. Both children and adults are affected by cancer. You may even know someone who is battling this disease. It is important to understand that knowledge is power. Knowledge of what may cause certain cancers enables medical researchers to design more effective treatment courses. And the more medical researchers understand about what causes various cancers, the closer they will come to finding cures.

The stories in this chapter all relate to the fight against cancer. In some instances, this means raising public awareness of the dangers of smoking, which can lead to diseases such as lung cancer. In others, it means raising money to fund important clinical and scientific research.

FIGHTING
CANCER

★ *Linda Ellerbee* ★

For 25 years, Linda Ellerbee has been a highly respected journalist. She has written two best-selling books and has also written for and anchored CBS, ABC, CNN, and NBC news shows for adults. Many kids enjoy Ellerbee's "Nick News" program on Nickelodeon. Through her company, Lucky Duck Productions, she produces, writes, and hosts this award-winning show.

In February 1992, Ellerbee was diagnosed with breast cancer. In true reporter fashion, she gathered every book and article she could find on the subject. With aggressive medical and surgical treatment, she was able to recover and continue working. Since that time, Ellerbee has dedicated herself to raising public awareness about breast cancer. In September 1993, she produced an ABC special based on her personal story. The show was called "The Other Epidemic: What Every Woman Needs to Know About Breast Cancer." Ellerbee said, "We are very candid on this show. We show you what a scar looks like and what reconstruction looks like....We say, 'Look, most of us live, so get that lump checked.' But we also say, 'Look how many of us are dying. Raise your voice.'"

Ellerbee frequently does public service announcements for a variety of hospitals and cancer organizations, such as the American Cancer Society. She also gives speeches about breast cancer without charging fees. Ellerbee is a member of the honorary board of Gilda's Club, which is a support center for people who have cancer and for their families. In April 1992, just two months after being diagnosed with cancer, Ellerbee spoke at a Gilda's Club function.

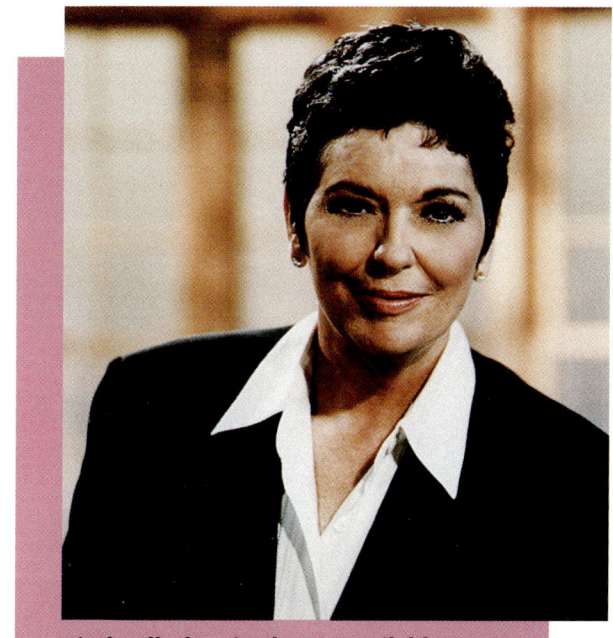

Linda Ellerbee is always available to educate people about cancer.

Ellerbee is very proud of the work she has done to bring the issue of cancer to the attention of children. She has worked to help them not be afraid. And Ellerbee has helped children cope when they or someone they know has been diagnosed with cancer. In an interview with *Coping* magazine she said, "Unless you make 'cancer' a scare word, to [children] it's not. We have done a number of stories having to do with cancer...stories where kids have had cancer...stories where their parents have had cancer...stories where other kids at school have cancer and how you deal with it. We want to give them positive models of people living with cancer. Not dying with it. Living with it." Ellerbee is a model of courage and determination. In the face of a life-threatening illness, she chose to fight for herself and to reach out to others.

★ *Richard Karn* ★

Richard Karn, who is the co-star of the hit comedy "Home Improvement," established the Richard Karn Star Days Foundation in 1994. Karn's non-profit organization produces an annual celebrity golf tournament benefit. The proceeds go to both a prominent cancer research center and the hospital that cared for Karn's mother, Louise Wilson, who died from cancer. After his mother's death, Karn decided to create this ongoing benefit for cancer research in her memory.

The research center that benefits from Karn's celebrity tournament is the Fred Hutchinson Cancer Research Center, an internationally known leader in cancer research. It trains scientists all over the world and is dedicated to eliminating cancer as a major cause of death. Overlake Hospital Medical Center, which also benefits from the tournament, is a top-notch hospital, providing comprehensive treatment to patients with cancer and other illnesses. In a 1995 interview with *People* magazine, Karn said about his mother's death, "I thought my parents were invincible. It never occurred to me she would die." Funds from the first celebrity golf tournament established the Louise Wilson Memorial Endowment for Oncology at Overlake Hospital. (Oncology is the study of tumors.)

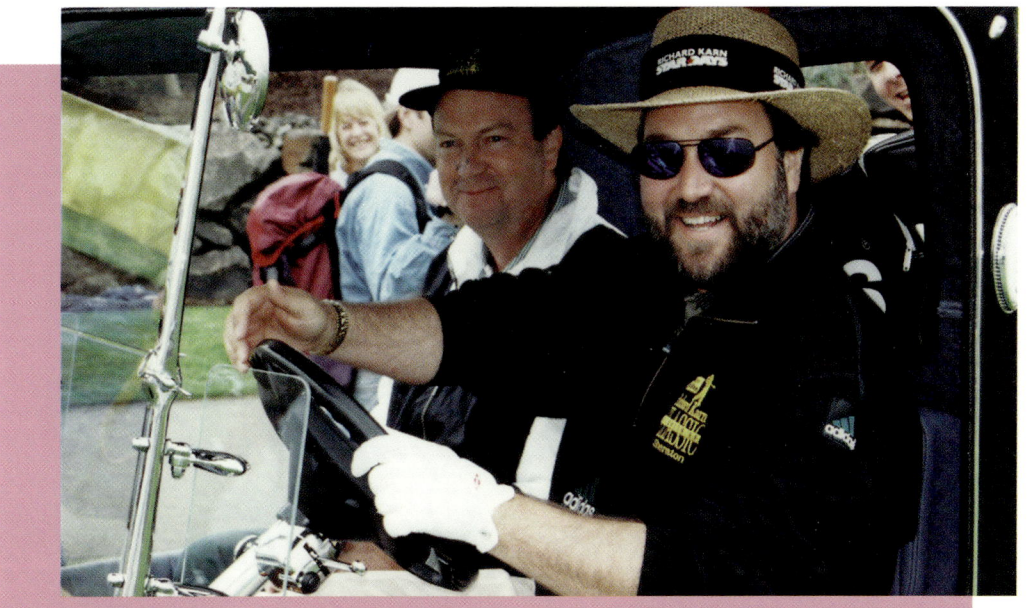

Richard Karn gives Bert Bennett, president of Wayne-Dalton, a ride at Karn's celebrity Golf Classic.

Wayne-Dalton, the world's largest garage-door manufacturer, is the corporate sponsor for Karn's annual gala. Karn became the spokesperson for this company after "Home Improvement" became a hit. With Wayne-Dalton's help, 100 percent of the profits from Richard Karn Star Days is donated to the two medical facilities.

Each year, dozens of celebrities gather to help Karn put on a star-studded weekend. In 1996, in addition to the golf tournament, celebrities donated their time to perform in a jazz concert, a comedy benefit, a baseball classic, a Planet Hollywood silent auction, and more. Carol Alt, Samuel Jackson, Casey Sander, Sharon Lawrence, Nicholas Turturro, Joe Regalbuto, Ken Ober, Kevin Costner, Bill Murray, Leslie Nielsen, and many, many other stars participated in these events.

The Star Days event, which was covered by ESPN, CNN, "Entertainment Tonight," and "Good Morning America," raised hundreds of thousands of dollars for cancer research.

$$\bigstar \quad \textit{Larry Hagman} \quad \bigstar$$

Actor Larry Hagman, best known for his roles as Major Anthony Nelson on "I Dream of Jeannie," and J.R. Ewing on "Dallas," has been a celebrity activist for more than 15 years. He has contributed immensely to two national organizations—the American Cancer Society and the National Kidney Foundation.

From 1981 to 1992, Hagman served as the national chairman for the ACS's Great American Smokeout. Over the years, this event has helped millions of people quit smoking. By quitting for the day of the Smokeout, people prove to themselves that they have the willpower to quit forever. The Great American Smokeout is open to teenagers as well as adults. Teenagers are encouraged to sign a pledge that they will lead smoke-free lives. In exchange for this pledge, they receive discount coupons for retail stores. Hagman has produced several public service announcements for the Smokeout. He has featured his mother—the famous actress Mary Martin—and Dr. C. Everett Koop, who is the former U.S. surgeon general.

In August 1995, Hagman began what he calls "the dawning of my second chance at life." He received a life-saving liver transplant that took 16 hours to perform. After it was over, Hagman said he had been given not only the gift of a healthy liver, but also the inspiration to make the rest of his life better—for himself and for others. Hagman often volunteers at St. Vincent's Hospital in Los Angeles. He visits transplant patients and offers them comforting advice. "I counsel, encourage, meet them when they come in for their operations, and after. . . . I try to offer some solace, like 'Don't be afraid, it will be a little uncomfortable for a brief time, but you'll be OK,'" he said in an Associated Press interview.

In addition to his local efforts at the hospital, Hagman is now the national chairman of the TransAction Council and

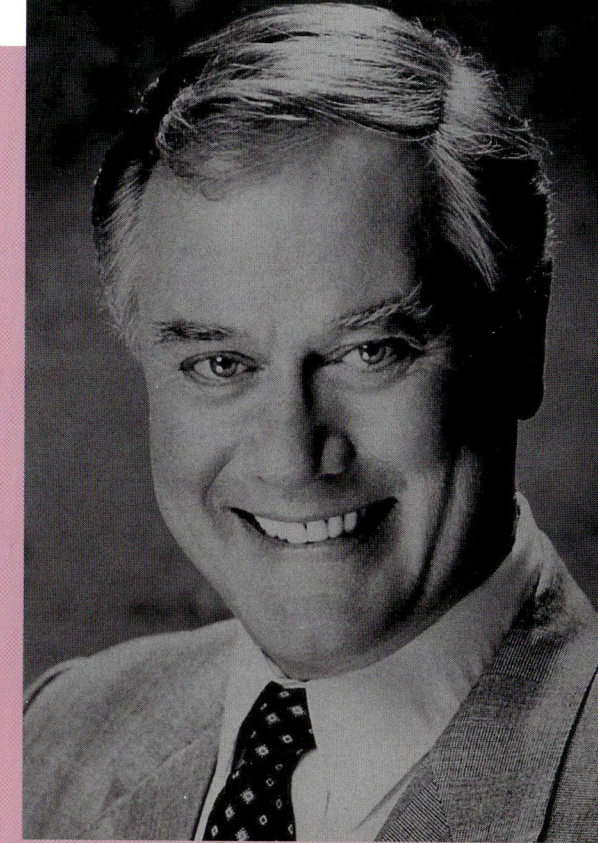

Larry Hagman has been helping people quit smoking for many years.

the national spokesperson for the National Kidney Foundation's Transplant Games. This is an Olympic-style athletic competition for people who have survived life-saving transplant operations—liver, heart, lung, kidney, pancreas, or bone marrow. In August 1996, almost 1,200 athletes competed in Salt Lake City, Utah, in events such as swimming, tennis, track and field, cycling, and basketball.

The Games began in 1982. The idea behind them is to change the public perception of people with transplants, and also to increase organ donation. Hagman told *USA Today*, "I hope my participation encourages more people to sign organ donor cards so that others can be given the same gift I've been lucky enough to receive." Adults who sign organ donor cards pledge that if they die suddenly, in an automobile accident for example, their organs can be donated to those in need of transplants.

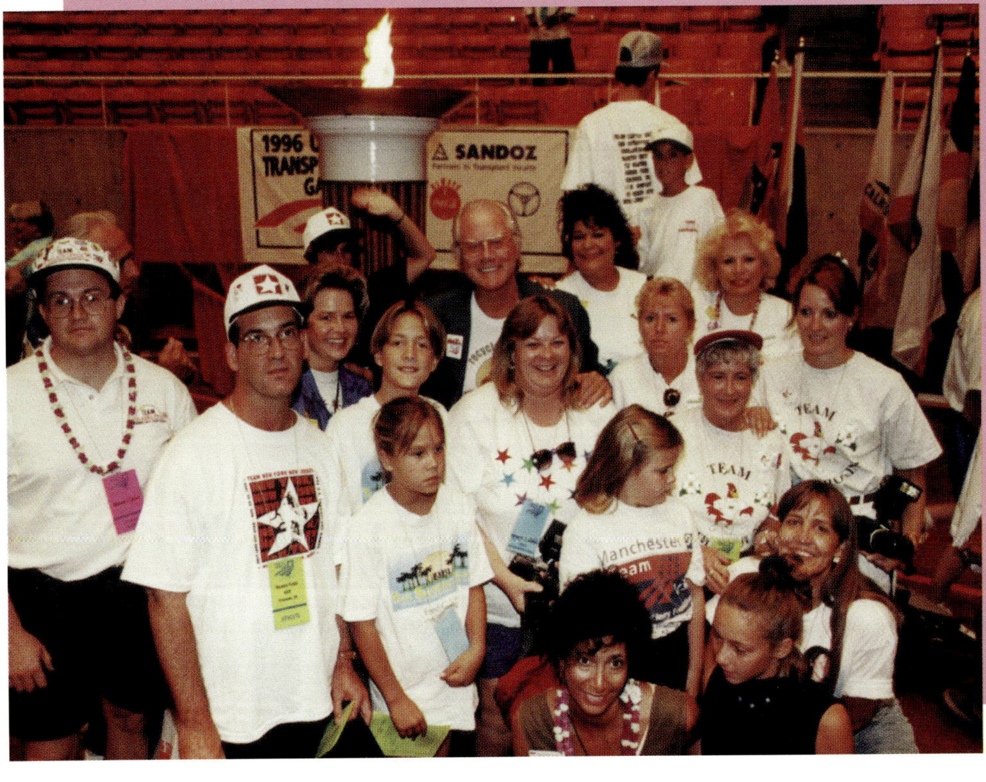

Larry Hagman (back row, center) poses with team members from the 1996 Transplant Games.

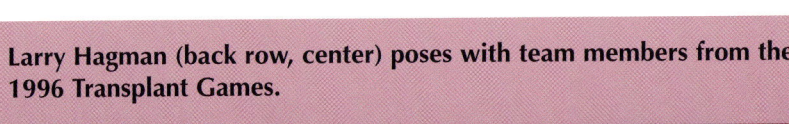

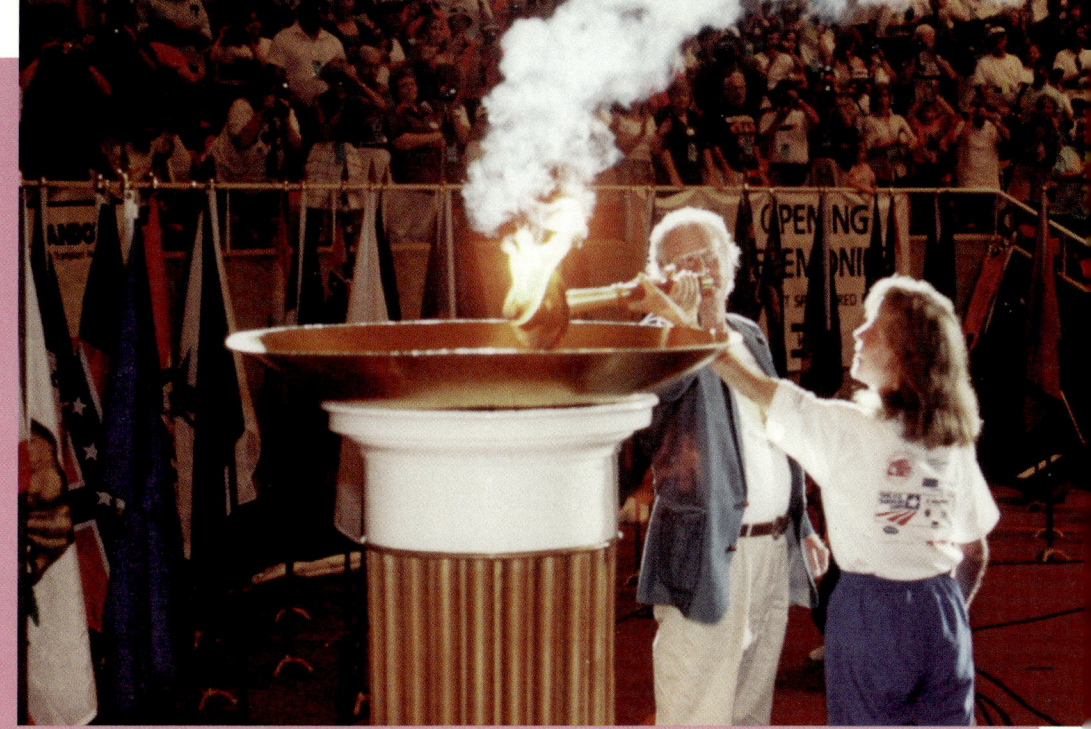

Larry Hagman and Maureen Olivero light the torch at the opening ceremony of the 1996 Transplant Games.

In addition to Hagman's participation, two other celebrities were involved as honorary spokespersons for the Transplant Games—Henry "Hank" Aaron, and Carl Lewis. Both of these professional athletes have been touched by this cause. Aaron and Lewis have both released organ donor cards designed to look like baseball cards through the Mickey Mantle Foundation. Lewis created the Wendy Marx Foundation for Organ Donor Awareness in an effort to increase the number of organs donated per year.

Hagman kicked off the 1996 Transplant Games by lighting the torch with Maureen Olivero, the Best Female Athlete of the 1994 Games. He also presented medals to competition winners throughout the event. In an August 1996 interview on "CBS This Morning," Hagman said of his motivation to volunteer, "I think it's very important to distribute your love and compassion around. That's the fun part of life now."

OTHER

MEDICAL

PROBLEMS

In addition to cancer and AIDs, there are many diseases and other medical problems that afflict millions of people throughout the world. Some of these health crises include heart disease, mental illness, Parkinson's disease, paralysis, liver disease, and hepatitis. There are literally thousands of causes for people to dedicate themselves to—and every one of them is worthwhile.

The celebrities in this chapter are all doing ongoing work that will benefit people for years to come. Their dedication and compassion for others can be contagious. They raise the public's awareness about these medical problems. And they encourage people to contribute the time and financial help that are needed to make a difference.

★ *Mandy Patinkin* ★

Mandy Patinkin is an actor, a singer, and a life-long activist with an enormous heart. He won an Emmy Award for his work on the television series "Chicago Hope" and a Tony Award for his performance in the Broadway musical *Evita*. Patinkin has been in numerous movies and Broadway productions. He also tours the United States, giving solo concerts to sold-out crowds.

Since he was a young man growing up in Chicago, Patinkin has helped others. From his parents, he learned the tradition of *tzedakah* (sah-DAH-kah) the Hebrew word for "charity," or "responsibility toward others." He recalls, "My parents were always very active in charities, and I just learned as a little kid how important it was." As an adult, the pace of his efforts accelerated in 1989, when his concert tours became popular. "Once I started the music, all these requests started coming to do benefits for every kind of charity in the world. . . . Peace projects, medical projects, political projects. So I would choose." And choose he has. Patinkin has donated his talents and countless hours of his time to benefit many different organizations.

Patinkin's work for the Crohn's and Colitis Foundation, which supports research on Crohn's disease and colitis—two inflammatory bowel diseases—began in 1989. (Inflammatory bowel diseases affect the large and small intestines.) He became involved with this group because his sister has suffered from Crohn's disease since she was 16. Whenever he gives a concert in an area where the foundation has a chapter, a group of benefit tickets are sold. Proceeds from these benefit tickets are donated to the organization. At a gathering after one of these concerts, Patinkin usually speaks about the progress that medical research has made on inflammatory bowel disease. Patinkin has also had a long history with Gilda's Club, an organization that offers emotional support to cancer patients and their families. He was one of the founding members, and he continues to do fund-raisers for Gilda's Club whenever the group needs him.

Another group that Patinkin is dedicated to is the Big Apple Circus Clown Care Unit. Since 1985, this community outreach program of the Big Apple Circus, in New York City, has been training clown "doctors." These "doctors" bring laughter and joy to hospitalized children, as well as to their parents and care-givers. Patinkin says of the group, "They go in to make the kids not be afraid of the common practices that go on in a hospital—a needle that is frightening to a child is turned into a whistle. They take a stethoscope, put it in bubbles, take the ends that go in your ears and put them in their mouth, and blow bubbles. They do all kinds of fun things with these kids who are going to have major procedures. And I was very moved by this." Patinkin was able to convince the people from "Chicago Hope" to write an episode featuring the Clown Care Unit. In doing so, Patinkin brought this extraordinary group to the attention of millions of

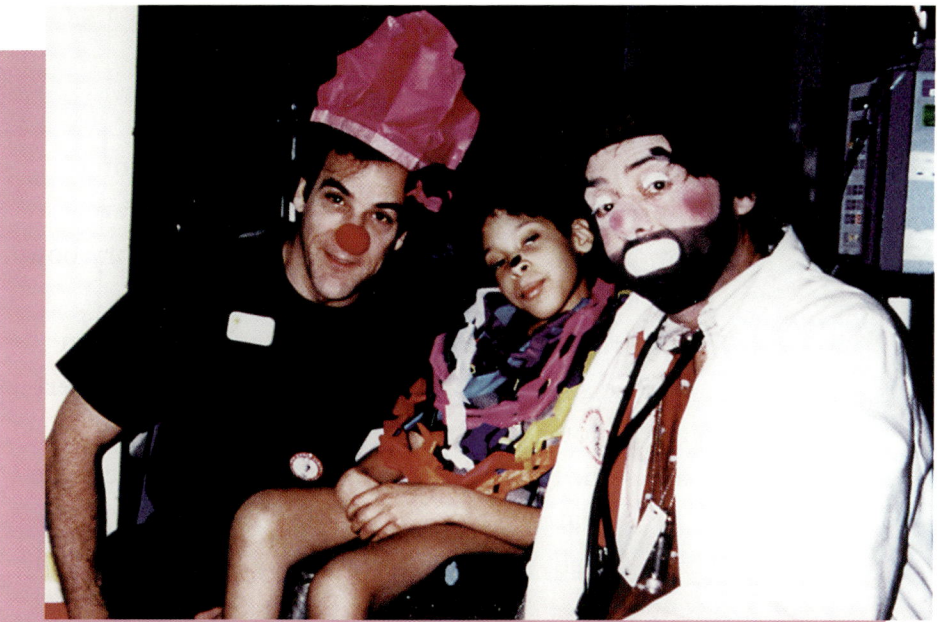

Mandy Patinkin (left) volunteers for the Big Apple Circus Clown Care Unit to bring joy to hospitalized children.

television viewers. Since then, he has been involved with the Clown Care Unit's efforts to make their program available to hospitals across the nation.

Patinkin's newest project is a nonprofit company called Tzedakah that he and his wife, Kathryn Grody, established in January 1997. Their company enables Patinkin to organize his own benefit concerts and choose the benefactors. On March 1, 1997, he began an 18-concert run at the Lyceum Theater in New York City that benefited five charities. They were the Crohn's and Colitis Foundation; the Association to Benefit Children (ABC), an advocacy group with temporary housing and programs for needy children all over New York; Physicians for Human Rights, which sends doctors to places like Bosnia and Rwanda; the National Dance Institute; and Peace Now, an organization dedicated to peace in the Middle East. Every cent of the profits from the concerts was donated to these five groups.

A SEVENTH GRADER INTERVIEWS MANDY PATINKIN

Question: After all these years of helping people in need, how do you feel?
Answer: Well, it's a great, great feeling. I try to teach my kids the same lesson. It's the best feeling, because if business has been good to me, it's good to give some back, and I give back as much as I can.

Q: How do you teach your kids about charity?
A: We do it by walking on the street, and you see a homeless person, and my kids give them some money in their pocket. We do it at the holiday season. We go and clean out all our toys, because we have too much. And we give all the toys to charities. We also buy new toys for some places....We have taught our kids from the beginning that in their allowance they get a certain amount of money, and that part of it goes to saving for school, and part of it goes to charities...the charities of their choice. So giving is a very important thing in our family. And my desire is to send that message out to the public and say, "find your way of giving, whatever it is."

Q: What kind of message do you want to get out to kids?
A: I'd like to get two messages out to kids. In terms of charities, always think of and never forget those who have less than you. And find a way to help balance out the world so that it is not so unfair that some have so much and some

Patinkin hopes that he will be able to make these concerts annual events and would like to choose different charities each year. He prefers to target organizations that don't have a lot of financial assistance from major corporations—groups that can really benefit significantly from his help. He says, "The message

have so little. Everyone someday should have a place to eat, a place to live, and a way to afford to enjoy some of the pleasures of this world. And the other thing is to follow your heart. Don't let anyone ever tell you that you can't do something that you think you can. Don't let anyone ever tell you that something is impossible . . . and experiment.

Danny Milano is a seventh grader at the Bailey Middle School in West Haven, Connecticut.

Mandy Patinkin shares his feelings about the importance of charity with Danny Milano.

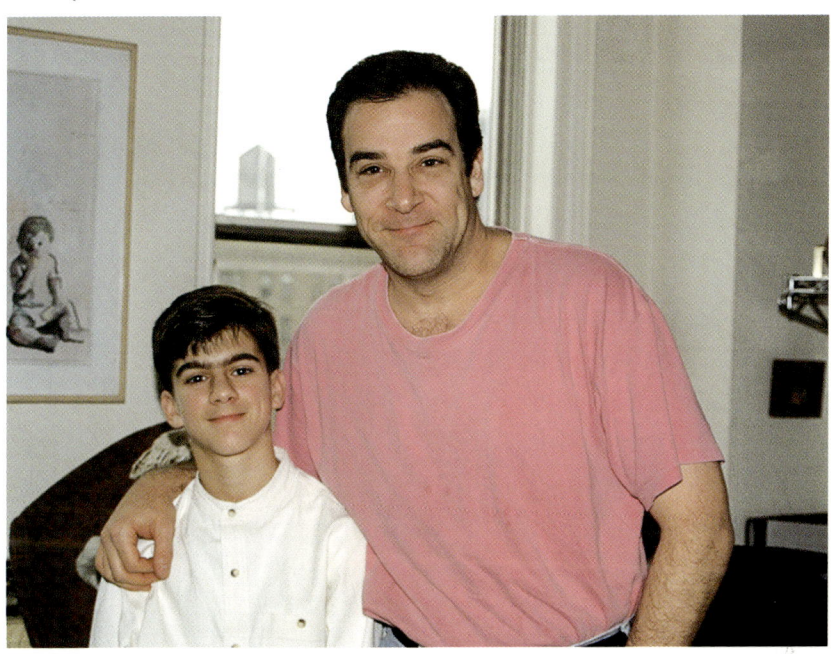

is not to try to raise a million dollars for each organization, but to give what you can. And so anybody out there who has done well enough in their life for that fiscal year . . . can take a little time out, and find a way to give something back. That's my point. It doesn't have to be thousands of dollars, it can be ten dollars."

★ Muhammad Ali and the National Parkinson Foundation ★

Muhammad Ali has been a champion for more than 35 years. He became internationally known when he won the gold medal for boxing at the Rome Olympics. He went on to become heavyweight champion three times and has called himself "The Greatest." Ali has proven himself to be the greatest, both in and out of the ring.

More than ten years ago, Ali was diagnosed with Parkinson's disease. This is a neurological illness that affects muscle control. It progresses slowly. As time goes on, patients lose more and more control over their muscle functions. The cause of the disease is unknown. Medical researchers do know, however, that the disease is related to an inadequate amount of a chemical in the brain called dopamine. About 1.5 million people in the United States are afflicted with Parkinson's disease.

The National Parkinson Foundation (NPF) was founded in 1957. This organization is dedicated to researching the cause of, and cure for, this disease. It also provides services and education to patients, family members, and caregivers. Muhammad Ali became the national spokesperson for this foundation in January 1996. In September 1996, Ali and the NPF began a public awareness campaign for the disease. Called

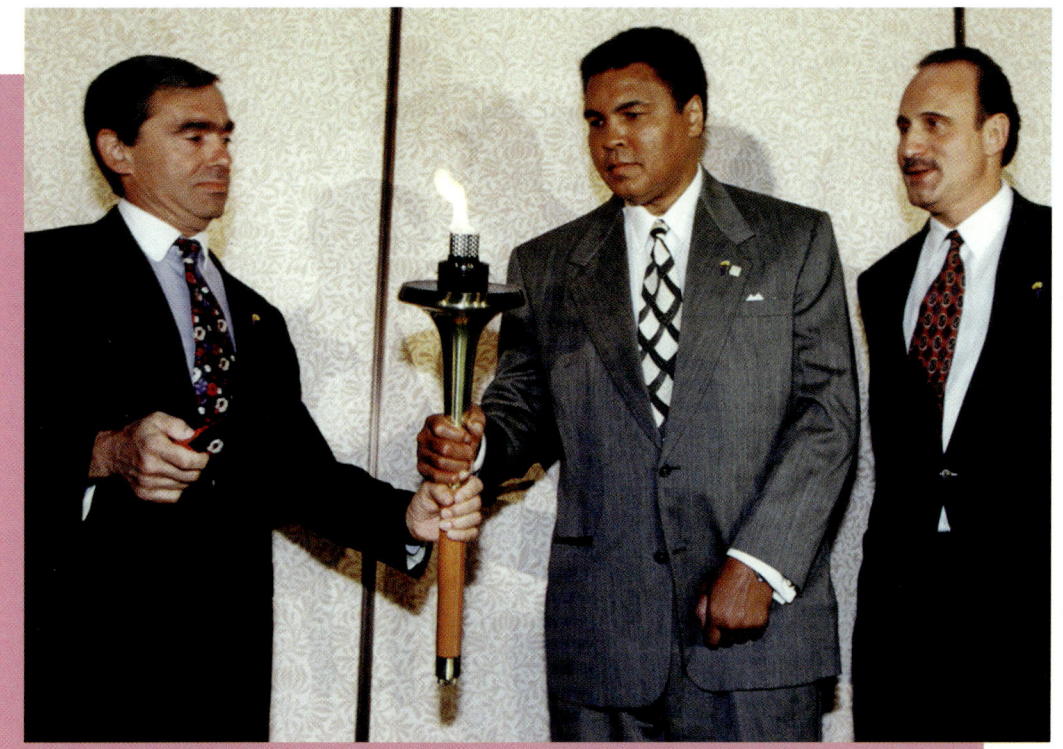

Muhammad Ali (center) dedicates the NPF's first "Fighting Flame" to kick off the Blazing Towards a Cure campaign.

Blazing Towards a Cure, the campaign uses the symbol of a flaming torch to light the way in finding a cure for Parkinson's disease.

When a slow-moving Ali with a trembling hand lit the torch to kick off the 1996 Olympics in Atlanta, Georgia, the world witnessed the strength of this champion. Then in September, Ali ignited the NPF's "Fighting Flame" for Parkinson's disease. The flame was lit at 45 NPF centers around the world in 1997. Ali was there to dedicate many of the centers.

Ali's wife, Lonnie, frequently speaks about her role as Ali's caregiver. Together they have brought hope to Parkinson patients everywhere. Ali will be the national spokesperson for the NPF for the next two years, dedicating his time to NPF events throughout the country.

The Larry King Cardiac Foundation

Larry King is one of the most famous interviewers of our time—he has interviewed more than 35,000 people! His award-winning show, "Larry King Live," has been on the air since 1985. King continues to inform and entertain viewers with celebrity interviews and political debates.

In 1988, after suffering from heart disease, Larry King had cardiac (heart) surgery that saved his life. Soon after, he founded the Larry King Cardiac Foundation so that heart patients in need of surgery would be able to receive the life-saving medical help that they must have. This nonprofit foundation aids people who are not able to afford adequate health insurance.

In the United States, someone has a heart attack every 20 seconds. Unfortunately, many people cannot afford good health care. Hospitals around the country have therefore agreed to work with King's foundation. Surgeons who operate on foundation patients do so at cost, which means that the hospital is only reimbursed for the materials that are used. The Larry King Cardiac Foundation is funded by annual fund-raising events and the profits from King's many books and public appearances.

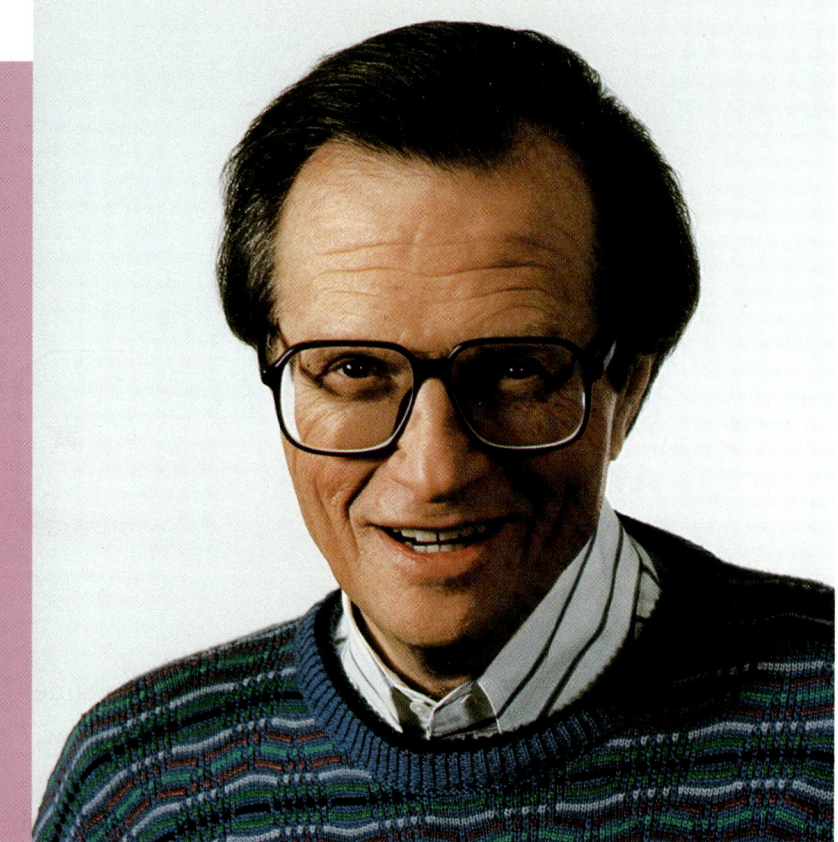
Larry King founded his cardiac foundation to help those who can't afford necessary heart surgery.

In addition to his foundation, King is a member of the Honorary Committee for the National Coalition for Heart and Stroke Research. This is a group of 15 medical organizations that are all dedicated to research and to the care of people who have experienced heart disease and strokes. Among these organizations are the American Heart Association, the American College of Cardiology, and the National Stroke Association. The coalition was created to increase public awareness of these diseases and to provide funding for the organizations. Through his generosity and dedication, Larry King has helped to save the lives of hundreds of people.

★ *Christopher Reeve* ★

In May 1995, Christopher Reeve, the actor made famous for his role as Superman, suffered severe injuries when he was thrown from his horse in a riding accident. The fall damaged his spinal cord. As a result, he was paralyzed from the neck down. It was a tragic accident, but Reeve rallied with amazing courage and strength. In the months that followed, Reeve had surgery and painful rehabilitation sessions. He is determined to walk again. Throughout this ongoing process, Reeve always appears to be cheerful and full of hope, as does his family. He has also found a way to help other paralysis patients.

Reeve has always been an activist. He has dedicated himself in the past to organizations such as Save the Children, Amnesty International, the National Resources Defense Council, America's Watch, People for the American Way, and The Creative Coalition (TCC). Reeve was one of the founding members of TCC and served as its president for many years. The organization works on behalf of social and political issues such as gun control, health care reform, and the environment.

But Reeve's most recent cause is a result of his personal experience. In September 1996, it was announced that the Reeve–Irvine Research Center would be opened at the University of California, Irvine (UCI).

Scientists at this center will be dedicated to searching for a cure for paralysis and other effects of spinal cord and brain disorders. The center is a collaborative effort between Christopher Reeve, philanthropist Joan Irvine Smith, UCI, and the American Paralysis Association.

According to the American Paralysis Association, about 250,000 Americans suffer from paralysis resulting from spinal cord injuries. Paralysis patients face lives of both physical and financial hardship. The people involved with the Reeve–Irvine Research Center hope to alleviate some of this by developing advances in this field. The creation of the Christopher Reeve Research Medal is just one effort of the center. This $50,000 award will be presented each year to a leading scientist doing spinal cord injury research. Christopher Reeve presented this award to the first recipient, Martin E. Schwab, in September

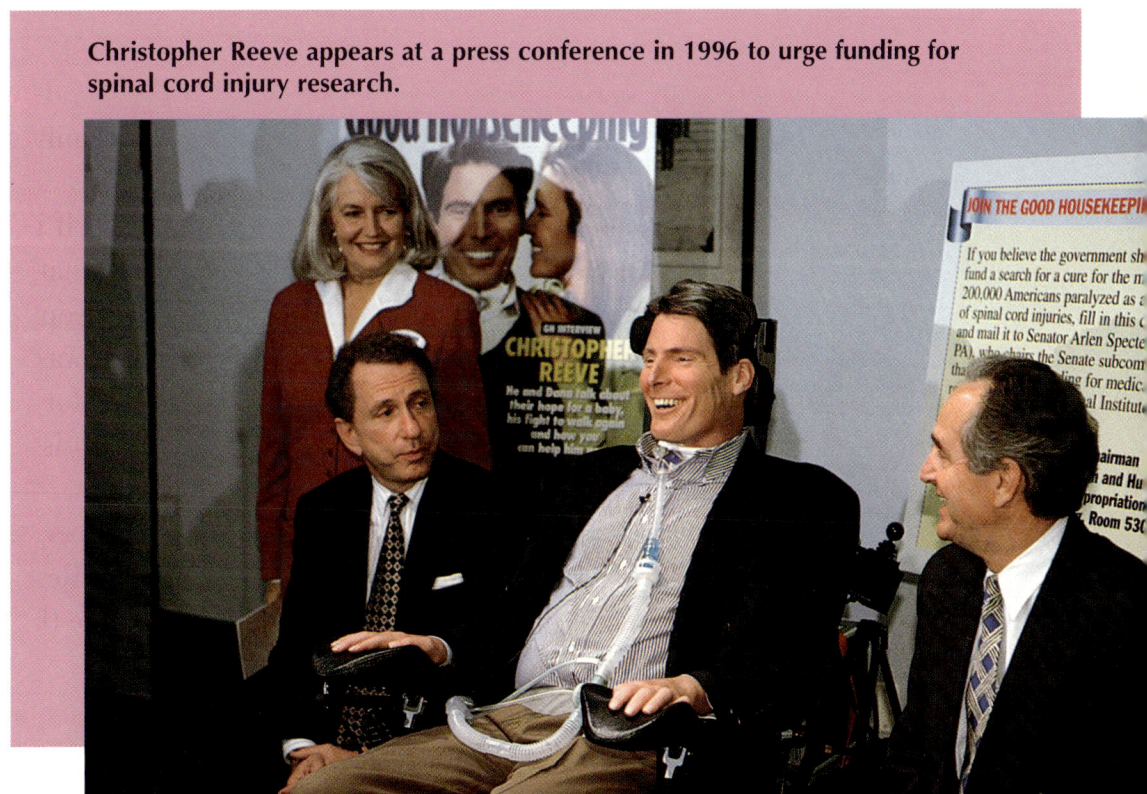

Christopher Reeve appears at a press conference in 1996 to urge funding for spinal cord injury research.

1996. The award money, along with $1 million for the center, was donated by Joan Irvine Smith.

Reeve says he views "this research effort and this program as a prototype [model] for future research centers worldwide. It is a critical step in the strategic plan to coordinate all spinal cord research efforts." His ongoing involvement with the center includes hosting fund-raising events with his wife Dana and Smith. Two different events raised $500,000 for the center. At one fund-raiser, a ten-year-old quadriplegic named Trent McGee had a dream come true when he and "Superman" talked together about dealing with their disabilities. Other celebrities, including Robin Williams, Jane Seymour, Joan Rivers, Lea Thompson, Ted Danson, and Mary Steenbergen, have attended events for the center to show their support.

At the beginning of 1996, in a separate effort, work began on establishing the Christopher Reeve Foundation. The foundation has two main missions—to help disabled people learn how to improve the quality of their lives and to raise money for spinal cord research. Money that is raised for spinal cord research will be used to fund research grants awarded by the American Paralysis Association. The first major fund-raiser for the Christopher Reeve Foundation took place on January 12, 1997, at the McCarter Theater in Princeton, New Jersey. A benefit concert was given, showcasing Mary Chapin Carpenter, Mandy Patinkin, Carly Simon, and John Lithgow—who all donated their talents to the event. The evening raised $300,000 for the new foundation.

Christopher Reeve's philanthropic efforts throughout his life have been significant. He is a shining example that a giving spirit cannot be daunted by even the most traumatic physical setback. He is truly an exceptional "Superman."

★ *Naomi Judd* ★

Country music star Naomi Judd has had a very strong affiliation with the American Liver Foundation (ALF) for several years. The ALF is dedicated to preventing, treating, and curing hepatitis and liver and gallbladder diseases through education and research. These diseases affect 25 million Americans.

Judd's interest in this organization is a personal one. After Naomi was diagnosed with a hepatitis virus, she stopped performing with her daughter Wynona Judd. Hepatitis is a virus and it is the main cause of liver disease in the United States. Approximately 15,000 people a year die of chronic viral hepatitis. To help the ALF in their efforts to fund research, Naomi Judd acts as the national spokesperson for this organization. In addition, she volunteers her time to many ALF events.

In 1993, Judd contributed $90,000 toward the establishment of the Naomi Judd Liver Scholar Awards. These awards are given to researchers of liver and gallbladder diseases. Dr. Karl P. Houglum from the University of California at San Diego was the recipient of the 1993 award. After winning this award Houglum said, "I spoke to Naomi Judd for 45 minutes, explaining my research with chronic active hepatitis. She was very interested because she is personally affected."

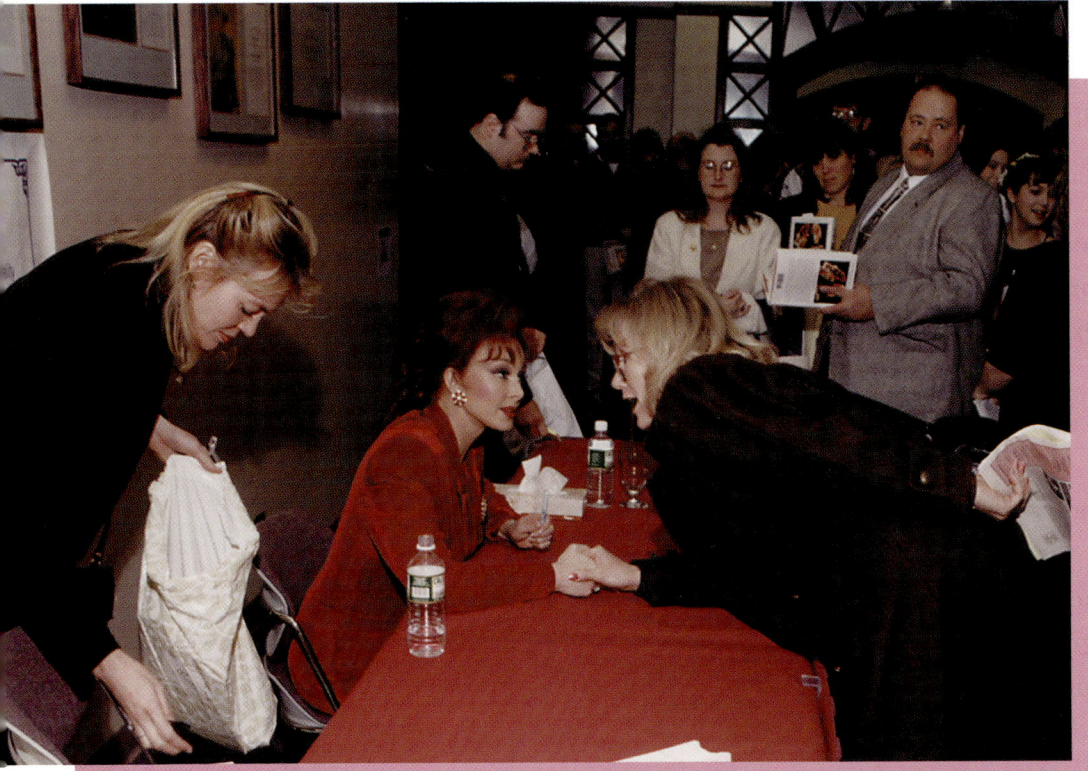

Naomi Judd talks with an audience member at one of her many speaking engagements where she educates the public about hepatitis.

In April 1993, Judd received the American Liver Foundation's Distinguished Service Award for her dedication to funding research efforts and educating the public about hepatitis. In April 1996, she was mistress of ceremonies at an annual Toys "R" Us benefit, which raised $2.8 million for 18 different children's health-care charities. She and Toys "R" Us also donated $100,000 to create the ALF's first Pediatric Liver Disease Research Award.

Judd appears in an ALF educational video for patients in which she discusses how viral hepatitis changed her life. She has given many interviews that highlight what she has learned about the disease. As a guest on "Oprah," she spoke of ALF's important work in front of millions of viewers. In addition, Judd has made two public service announcements for the American Liver Foundation. Judd's philanthropic work for the ALF has greatly promoted awareness of hepatitis and liver diseases. Her work as national honorary spokesperson will continue over the next several years.

★ ★

The celebrities that you have read about in this book have all made enormous contributions to a great variety of causes. Each one has dedicated his or her time with the hope of making a significant difference in the lives of many people. They have fought to further research, brightened the outlook for sick children, supported adequate health care for those who cannot afford it, and promoted prevention and education services. They are all exceptional role models who believe that anyone can initiate change if they believe in something strongly enough. We thank them for their admirable efforts.

Glossary

activist A person who believes in, and actively supports, a cause.

cardiac Relating to the heart.

cerebral palsy A disorder that is characterized by a lack of control over the muscles, resulting from damage to the brain before or during birth.

cystic fibrosis An inherited disease that affects the ducts of certain glands. It often affects the pancreas and lungs.

diabetes A disease that is characterized by a deficiency of insulin and a resulting excess of sugar in the blood.

insulin A hormone that regulates the body's use and storage of sugar and other carbohydrates.

legislation The making or passing of laws.

leukemia A disease characterized by the formation of abnormal numbers of white blood cells.

metabolism The biological and chemical processes that occur in a living being.

muscular dystrophy A disease that is characterized by a gradual weakening of the muscles. There are nine different types of this disease.

nonprofit A group or organization that is not operating in order to make a profit.

pediatrician A doctor who specializes in the branch of medicine that deals with children and babies.

philanthropy The giving of money or time in order to benefit a cause.

reconstruction To rebuild something. In the context of breast cancer, reconstruction can refer to surgery relating to the loss of a breast.

Further Reading

Bergman, Thomas. *One Day at a Time: Children Living with Leukemia.* Ada, OK: Gareth Stevens, 1989.

Chandler, Gary and Kevin Graham. *Celebrity Activists: Environmental Causes.* New York: Twenty-First Century Books, 1997.

Hawkes, Nigel. *Medicine and Health.* New York: Twenty-First Century Books, 1994.

Huggins, Nathan. *Whoopi Goldberg: Entertainer.* New York: Chelsea House, 1995.

Landau, Elaine. *Understanding Cancer.* New York: Twenty-First Century Books, 1994.

Finn, M., and Jerry Lewis, intro. *Mary Tyler Moore: The Award-Winning Actress Who Has Diabetes.* New York: Chelsea House, 1995.

Manning, Karen. *AIDS.* New York: Twenty-First Century Books, 1996.

Richardson, Wendy and Jack Richardson. *Entertainers: Through the Eyes of Artists.* Chicago, IL: Childrens Press, 1991.

For More Information

American Cancer Society
1599 Clifton Road, N.E.
Atlanta, GA 30329
Website: http://www.cancer.org/

Muscular Dystrophy Association
National Headquarters
3300 East Sunrise Drive
Tucson, AZ 85718-3208
Website: http://www.mdausa.org/

American Heart Association
1150 Connecticut Avenue, N.E.
Suite 810
Washington, DC 20036
Website: http://www.amhrt.org/

St. Jude Children's Research Hospital
501 St. Jude Place
Memphis, TN 38105-1942
Website: http://www.stjude.org/

National Parkinson Foundation, Inc.
1501 N.W. 9th Avenue, Bob Hope Road
Miami, FL 33136-1494
Website: http://www.parkinson.org/

Index

Photo Credits

Page 8: Courtesy of Newman's Own, Inc.; pages 11, 12: Courtesy of the Muscular Dystrophy Association; page 14: Courtesy of Starlight Children's Foundation International; pages 16, 17: Courtesy of St. Jude Children's Research Hospital; page 19: Courtesy of the Juvenile Diabetes Foundation; page 21: ©Kevin Mazur 1996; page 22: Clint Steib; pages 24, 25: Courtesy of the Elton John AIDS Foundation; pages 27, 53: Photofest; pages 28, 55: ©Martin Simon/SABA; page 30: Billy Bytsura, 1996/Courtesy of AmFAR; page 33 (upper left): Photofest; page 33 (upper right): ©V. Vlamos/REA/SABA; page 33 (lower left): Steve Starr/SABA ©1995; page 33 (lower right): Craig Sjodin/ABC/Photofest; page 37: Courtesy of Lucky Duck Productions; page 39: Courtesy of Richard Karn Star Days; pages 41, 42, 43: Courtesy of the National Kidney Foundation; page 47: Courtesy of Babies & Children's Hospital of New York, Virginia C. Keim, and Mandy Patinkin; page 49: ©Laurie Foster; page 51: Courtesy of the National Parkinson Foundation's new public awareness campaign; page 58: ©John Sinclair, Master Photographer.